How to Keep Your Loved One Safe in a Nursing Home

A Quick Reference Guide

Andrew D. Weinberg, M.D., FACP

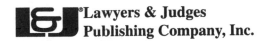
Lawyers & Judges
Publishing Company, Inc.

**Lawyers & Judges
Publishing Company, Inc.**
P.O. Box 30040 • Tucson, AZ 85751-0040
(800) 209-7109 • FAX (800) 330-8795
e-mail: sales@lawyersandjudges.com

Library of Congress Cataloging-in-Publication Data

Weinberg, Andrew David.
   How to keep your loved one safe in a nursing home : a quick reference guide / Andrew D. Weinberg.
      p. cm.
   ISBN 1-930056-52-4 (pbk.)
   1. Nursing home patients. 2. Nursing homes. I. Title.
   RA997.W435 2003
   362.16--dc22

                                2003018313

ISBN 1-930056-52-4
10 9 8 7 6 5 4 3 2

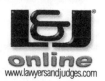
www.lawyersandjudges.com

Dedication

To all the nurses, doctors and other healthcare professionals who are involved in the nursing home industry. Your hard work and dedication will not be forgotten.

Contents

Chapter 1

Nursing Home Life: The Vital Statistics

During one of our weekly visits to my grandmother's tiny two room apartment, where she lived alone, we brought her a new novel she had told us she was eager to read. At our next visit the following weekend we noticed she had carefully placed a bookmark at the end of the first chapter. When we inquired about how she liked the book, she replied she was thrilled with it and couldn't wait to read more. The following week we noticed the bookmark was in exactly the same place. We asked her why she wasn't reading and she replied, obviously quite annoyed, that she read a chapter every single night. It soon became apparent to us that she was losing her memory and she could not remember she had finished the first chapter. Every night she would start the whole book over again, not realizing she had already read the first chapter multiple times. It was our first real definitive sign that she had Alzheimer's. Within six months, she could no longer cook or wash her clothes and she had lost significant weight. Soon afterwards, we made the terribly painful decision to put her in a nursing home. We all felt terribly guilty but knew, after a time, that we had made the right decision.

—Grandson of an Alzheimer's patient

If you are reading this book, one will assume you have made the extremely difficult and potentially guilt-ridden decision to place a loved one in a nursing home (nursing facility). This action is never without significant emotional and economic consequences. Although it is true that each person who resides in a nursing home (now referred to as a resident) is protected by state and federal regulations that he or she is entitled to receive quality care and have specific legal rights and privileges, the reality is that this just doesn't happen all the time. There are several excellent resources available on how to choose a nursing home which are listed in the reference section but this book will focus on the difficult task of monitoring the care your loved one receives in the facility you have chosen. This is an ongoing responsibility and the benefits of good oversight by the family should never be underestimated.

As you will not be surprised to know, there are many rules and regulations that govern how a nursing home should run. One of the more important ones you should have some familiarity with is called the federal Omnibus Budget Reconciliation Act (OBRA) of 1987 (and since revised by Congress a number of times) which listed, for the first time, national standards for care in nursing homes and outlined specific resident rights (see Appendix A). This Act is often called the "Nursing Home Reform Law." This law entitles the nursing home resident (or legal representative) to

1. receive pertinent information on all aspects of care and to participate in care-planning decisions,
2. make independent personal choices,
3. receive confidentiality in all aspects of financial issues and personal and medical care as well as receiving medical treatments in private,
4. be treated at all times with dignity and respect,
5. be protected against transfer out of the facility except for specific reasons and with a thirty-day notice,
6. raise any care concerns or complaints that must be responded to by the staff without any fear of retaliation, and
7. choose his or her own physician within the facility.

Many public advocate groups, such as the National Citizens' Coalition for Nursing Home Reform, believe that nursing home care in too many homes is mediocre at best. Of the approximately 19,000 nursing homes in this country, less than ideal care along with flaws in the monitoring and enforcement programs *can* result at times in bad outcomes for certain individuals. That is why you, the family member, must become an informed, motivated and involved individual to ensure that your loved one will receive the best possible care at all times in the nursing home you have selected. This is not an easy assignment and will require constant vigilance and follow-up. This book will provide you with the means to work with the nursing staff in a teamwork fashion and to know when, how and why you should bring your concerns and questions to those in charge.

This book is also organized in such a way that each chapter can stand on it own and it can be read in any order.

Anymore, there is hardly a month that goes by that some TV station or newspaper does not publish an "expose" of alleged horrible care or abuse at a local nursing home. Most of these stories are blown out of proportion and prey on the fears of the average American to expect the worse from any nursing home. This horrible care is the exception, not the rule, for most nursing homes in this country.

It is true, however, that there has been an avalanche of lawsuits during the last ten years against nursing home corporate owners, administrators, directors of nursing, medical directors and attending physicians for alleged lapses in care. The jury verdicts and settlements run into the hundreds of millions of dollars each year. This is not because the defense industry cannot find qualified attorneys to represent the staff working in these facilities, but that juries have clearly demonstrated a rising anger towards patterns of neglect, abuse and lapses in clinical care that many times could have been prevented by better communication and coordination of care. That is the goal of this book, to impart to you the "secret knowledge" to protect those you love from these lapses before they can cause harm. It will help you to sort out truly legitimate concerns from those that are not realistic expectations and how to advocate for your loved one by knowing how to confront the "system" and win. *You* can be the vital link to overseeing quality care for your relative involving dozens of professionals to whom access is often difficult and where frustration can be a daily occurrence.

Modern day nursing homes are the descendents of the old county "poor farms," where individuals who were no longer able to care for themselves were often physically dragged to by their children. Prior to these county establishments, which were generally poorly run and inadequately inspected, the children were responsible for taking care of their older, dependent parents. Society has changed. Even in Japan nowadays, where care of one's parents was always considered a sacred and honored duty, the advent of two working spouses has led to the establishment and utilization of quite a number of nursing homes, some of which are actually located in Europe due to the scarcity of available land on the Japanese mainland. A phrase that is often repeated in our country that "one mother can take care of four children but four children cannot take care of one mother." Nursing homes, for better or worse, have become an ingrained part of our culture and life in every state.

Our society and even Congress often express an archaic and negative attitude towards the older, frail and cognitively impaired individual and this cold, hard fact has remained one of our country's greatest challenges to overcome. The work, far from us not being able to see the light at the end of the tunnel, is more appropriately described as us not even having entered the tunnel at all! While the older, active eighty-year-old is still welcome in our society, the eighty-year-old with Alzheimer's is often shunned, not only by society but sometimes by certain family members as well. There is a real fear in this country of growing old and of looking old and the progressive loss of one's mind and functional abilities through the disease process of dementia is very threatening and often distasteful to some individuals.

In the vast and overwhelming array of federal and state regulations governing nursing homes (second only to the nuclear power industry in sheer number), the nursing home resident often seems to have the least authority or is given fewer opportunities to make personal decisions regarding care. Although cognitive impairment is the most common reason for an individual to enter a nursing home, it is not the only illness and one's mental function may remain relatively intact for sometime in a number of illnesses (e.g., Parkinson's disease). Thus, involving the resident in as many decisions as possible within the nursing home can help to make the transition somewhat less difficult. However, it is often up to the family to set the framework of care for their loved one, including consent for medication trials for certain behavioral issues, types of food, evaluation for new or ongoing medical problems, hospitalization for an acute illness and the degree to which resuscitation techniques should be carried out in the event of a cardiopulmonary event. The family is also usually responsible for advising the staff and attending physician of any Advance Directive information or "living will" that exists, as well as any pertinent medical history that is not available to the healthcare providers from other sources.

Understanding the primary goals for treatment and related psychosocial issues for your loved one in the nursing home is a critical first step. You must be prepared to spend time in the facility learning how the care patterns work and then being prepared to assist in adapting the facility's routine with the needs of your loved one. An example of this type of situation might involve a nursing home that routinely awakens their residents at 5 A.M. so that morning hygiene can be completed prior to breakfast being served. To someone used to sleeping late in the morning, this may lead to a somewhat harsh adjustment period. If your loved one protests against being gotten out of bed at an early hour, he may be subsequently labeled as "uncooperative" or "agitated" during morning care and the staff may then seek orders for medication to "calm" the resident down. Always investigate the care routines if you are informed that the staff has documented such undesirable "behaviors" and request an alteration in the care times if you believe this to be the cause of the "agitation."

Primary goals for care and facility support should include *at least* the following.

- There are adequate numbers of licenses nurses and certified nursing assistants (CNAs) present each day and on every shift to treat the resident in a timely manner. All residents are treated as an individual person, not as an "illness" or a "room number."
- Provision of adequate and varied food preparation (including temperatures that are appropriate to the food being served!) with the ability to provide for special food requests (unless medically contraindicated) by the resident.
- Dignity and respect shown to the residents at *all* times.
- Availability of varied and meaningful activities seven days a week through their activity department that adds to the quality of the resident's life (this does *not* mean placing residents in front of a television for hours at a time!).
- Medical staff assigned to the care of the resident who strive to stabilize all chronic medical conditions present and respond in a timely manner to all acute medical issues that arise.

Interestingly, the average physician in the United States knows surprising little of how long-term nursing home care works. It is estimated that approximately 85 percent of U.S. physicians never set foot again in a nursing home once they leave their formal medical training, unless it is as a patient themselves! Although there are about 8,000 physicians who have formally been certified as geriatricians (physicians who have special training and expertise in the care of the older adult), most of these physicians are hospital-based in academic centers and do not routinely care for those residing in local nursing homes.

The majority of medical care in nursing homes is actually provided by family practitioners or general internists, most of who also have busy general medical practices. The nursing home work by these practitioners is usually completed before or after their normal office hours and may be supplemented by the use of nurse practitioners or physician assistants. The average physician is only obligated to visit the residents living in nursing homes once every sixty days after a monthly visit for the first ninety days. It remains an ongoing challenge in this country to attract more highly motivated and well-trained physicians to work in the nursing home setting.

Some important statistics to remember about nursing homes

- Approximately 1.7 million residents live in 19,000 nursing homes in the U.S.
- At any given time approximately 5 percent of America's population lives in nursing homes.
- The majority of residents are female and eighty-five years or older.
- The primary reasons that someone is placed in a nursing home include his underlying medical condition, declining functional status, bowel incontinence and lack of appropriate family support or community-based home care.
- Most U.S. nursing homes (75 percent) are run for profit.
- Most facilities are typically staffed by one licensed practical nurse (LPN) for each twenty to thirty beds. Registered nurses (RNs) are generally only seen in the position of director of nursing, clinical supervisor or assigned to coding, functional documentation activities or Medicare/Medicaid billing responsibilities (see Chapter 2).
- Over 90 percent of the hands-on care for residents is provided by CNAs whose level of training is approximately only seventy-five hours. CNAs, overall, are generally poorly educated and paid low wages.

- Turnover rates for licensed nurses average approximately 45 percent per year and for CNAs the rate may be as high as 100 percent per year.
- Polypharmacy (too many prescribed medications at once) and the overuse of antipsychotic medications remain an ongoing challenge.
- Many medical conditions, such as chronic pain, depression and urinary incontinence remain misdiagnosed or untreated.
- As physicians are only required to visit every sixty days (after the required thirty-day visits for the first three months), on-site medical evaluation for acute problems is not routinely available.

The time you spend monitoring the care in a facility will not only reassure you that you are doing everything possible but will serve as a conduit for you to receive and give information to the nursing staff and attending physician. The ability to be able to communicate with the staff when an acute illness arises is a critical function and you should always leave multiple telephone numbers where you can be reached, especially when traveling outside of your home area.

Ten golden points to always remember

1. Guilt for placing someone in a nursing home will be laid on you either by your loved one themselves or by another relative. Adjust to it the best you can and focus on providing the best care you can arrange.
2. Talking to family members of other nursing home residents will immediately identify problem areas to watch out for in the facility.
3. Don't ever leave any valuables with your loved one in the facility. No matter how much these items may mean to the individual, if it has value it may get stolen or lost at some point. If you wish, you may bring the items for your loved one when you visit and take them back when you leave for safekeeping. You can also consider using cubic zirconium diamonds to substitute for real ones (if you use this option, let the staff know).
4. Always contact the attending physician directly by telephone after your loved one is admitted to a nursing home. The main office of the facility will be able to give you the number. If he or she doesn't call

you back within two business days (during the week), it's already time to change doctors! In an emergency, the nursing home can always reach your physician or the assigned covering physician (It's the law!).

5. If you don't understand a medication that has been ordered for your loved one, speak up to the nursing staff and question it. They can always get in touch with the physician to obtain an explanation for you. Remember, there are no stupid questions when it comes to nursing homes, especially when it relates to medication use.

6. Eat a meal at the facility. There is no better way to check the quality of the food being served than to eat a meal there yourself (you will probably be charged for the meal, this is a normal procedure). You may need to arrange for this in advance as the number of extra meals available for any given mealtime can be fairly tightly controlled in most facilities. Most importantly, monitor the food and fluid intake of your loved one on a regular basis. Poor nutrition and dehydration remain leading clinical problems for many residents of nursing homes, especially in the latter stages of dementia-type illnesses. Regularly ask for and follow the monthly weights, which are required to be obtained in all nursing homes in the United States. If the weight is declining for more than one month in a row, request that the dietitian be called to consult (a physician's order for this can be obtained by the nursing staff).

7. If the roommate sharing the room with your loved one is extremely loud and seems to be inappropriately matched, request a new roommate or a room change from the social services director. You have a right to request room changes although the availability of other rooms may be very limited at times.

8. Participate in the care planning conferences that are held on a regular basis (usually quarterly or more frequently as needed). Ask them to try to schedule these meetings at a time when you can attend or, if unable to be physically present, ask them to arrange a telephone speaker system to allow you to participate. These meetings review the care, physical assessments, medications and other issues that may be affecting the quality of life for your loved one in the facility. Be prepared to ask questions during the meeting if you have con-

cerns or send a written list of issues to the facility that you would like discussed at the meeting (see Chapter 4).

9. Always keep an eye on grooming issues. If your loved one does not appear to have had their hair combed, teeth brushed or have clean clothing on, find out why. Check to see if others in the facility have similar grooming problems. Speak to the director of nursing or administrator if you feel the staffing ratio is chronically inadequate to provide the necessary care for the number and medical condition of the residents living on that particular section of the facility (see Chapter 6). Ongoing dental care is also very critical for overall good health and the family should continue to schedule regular checkups and cleanings at the family's expense with your loved one's regular dentist. Quality dental care on-site at the nursing home is extremely rare to find.

10. If restraints are being requested or ordered, make sure the facility has tried alternative methods prior to their use. Restraints should be a last resort for someone in a facility as they can contribute to further decline in functional status (weakness of leg muscles due to decreased walking) or injury (full bed siderails being used). Make sure the nursing department has completed an assessment regarding the need and potential benefit of any restraint being recommended. Restraint use should be monitored on a regular basis and the least restrictive method used whenever possible. Regular review of the continued need for restraints is required by law and attempts at reduction in their use should be considered when clinically appropriate.

This chapter has set the tone for how intricate and challenging the nursing home structure can be and some of the major areas of care that will need to be monitored. This book will cover in detail the various areas reviewed in this chapter. The theme we will follow is that ongoing oversight, constructive comments and appropriate interventions can make a dramatic improvement in the care your loved one receives. Now, let's get to work!

Chapter 2

The Basics: Who Controls What in a Nursing Home

Those who manage don't understand how something should be done.
Those who understand how something should be done, don't manage.
—Old business proverb

The control of day-to-day operations of a nursing home may appear confusing to the casual observer. It is important for you to have an understanding of who controls what within a facility if you are to get what you need for your loved one. This chapter will take you through the hierarchy of command in a typical nursing home.

The nursing home's primary goal is to provide your loved one with the highest quality of care possible and this requires an interdisciplinary approach. The overall plan of care is coordinated by this team of health professionals and spells out in detail all interventions that will be followed. Descriptions of the key players in a nursing home follow.

Nursing Home Administrator

The administrator of a nursing home is responsible for the overall leadership of the facility and oversees all operational aspects of the facility. He or she may at times have a financial ownership in the building itself or may work for a management company that directs operations but does not own the building or the corporation that actually owns the business. For example, many not-for-profit corporations which own a number of facilities may hire a management team to work on site at these facilities and direct the day-to-day operations. However, any concerns regarding any aspect of the care or billing procedures that cannot be resolved at a lower administrative level should be directed to the administrator. These individuals typically wield the most power in any given facility.

Director of Nursing (DON)

The DON is responsible for the overall supervision of the nursing care and ensures that all medical orders are carried out by the staff. She or he is also often responsible for interviewing potential employee applicants, reviewing nursing work schedules and staff: patient ratios per shift, attending various committee meetings, liaison duties between the administrator, the medial director and staff and discussing unresolved care concerns with family members. She may also assist the Administrator in overseeing other healthcare professionals who work in the facility including the dietitian, physical, occupational and recreational therapists and social workers, environmental and maintenance workers and laundry personnel. All care-related issues will arrive on the DON's desk before they will reach the administrator as the DON reports to the administrator in the facility hierarchy. The DON typically coordinates the care with the individual nurse managers, charge nurses or supervisors in the facility.

If you have a concern regarding the environment, meals or the nursing care being delivered, you should first discuss it with the floor's day charge nurse or unit manager. Ultimately if you are unhappy with the response you obtain at this level, you should make an appointment to meet and discuss all unresolved issues with the DON. It is always best to do such meetings in person (see Chapter 7).

Medical Director

Each nursing home is required by federal regulation to have a physician medical director on contract with the facility. The number of hours that a medical director is physically in the building may vary from two hours weekly to almost daily visits for those with a full-time position within the nursing home. Full-time medical director positions, however, are very unusual.

The medical director performs an administrative role in the facility and does not involve the routine care of residents in the nursing home (that role is described under "physician" below). The medical director is usually assigned as the attending physician for those residents being admitted who will not have their community physician following their care after admission and he or she is also a member of various nursing home committees. Most importantly, the medical director must be available seven days a week for any emergencies in which the resident's regularly assigned physician cannot be reached. The medical director is also responsible for the overall delivery of medical care in the facility and deals with any care issues that might arise concerning any of the physicians caring for residents at the nursing home.

Physician

This is the assigned physician who is responsible for all medical care issues from the time of admission. A medical director may also be the physician for a number of the nursing home residents but this function represents an entirely different role. The medical director is often assigned by the facility as the attending physician when the family does not have any other physician selected to serve in this role.

Residents and their families have the right to select any physician they wish as long as that individual is licensed and can meet all of the requirements for becoming a staff physician at that particular facility. In reality, most physicians do not follow their patients into the nursing home but have one of the local nursing home physicians assume the care. All nursing home residents must be seen for an admission physical exam usually within three days of admission. (This rule can vary from state to state and from facility to facility.) Following the initial exam, the physician is required by federal regulations to visit monthly for the next three months. After this initial period the physician may then visit every sixty days if the clinical issues being monitored are stable.

The physician, however, must be available twenty-four hours a day, seven days a week for any emergencies or must arrange for a covering physician if he or she will be out of town and not reachable. If you notice that the physician does not return inquiries from you within a timely manner after calling his or her office directly, you should consider switching to another physician who may be more accessible.

Although required visits by the physician must be carried out in the nursing home, you may also arrange for consults outside of the facility with any physician in the community. Please be advised you will need to make the appointment yourself and arrange transportation at your own expense. Also, any new medication changes recommended by the consulting physician will need to be approved by the assigned nursing home physician as all medications given at the facility are ordered under this physician's name and license number. You may not bring any outside prescriptions in without the permission of the attending physician and only with the knowledge and agreement of the facility. Each facility has rules regarding the use of outside pharmacies other than the one that holds the current contract to provide such services to the nursing home.

You should always obtain the contact information for the physician at the time of admission. The nurses also know how to reach the physician in an emergency and you can always ask them to contact him or her if you feel that an acute medical change in your relative's condition warrants a call. You should not hesitate to insist on this if you feel uncomfortable with any acute change.

Nurse Practitioners (NPs) and Physician Assistants (PAs)

Physicians may have NPs or PAs assisting them in the day-to-day care of nursing home residents. Although many states allow NPs and PAs to write treatment and medication orders, the physician they work with is ultimately responsible for all of their orders. If a clinical issue arises that the NP or PA feels needs clarification, they would contact their supervising physician to discuss it with him or her.

Most NPs and PAs have excellent communication skills and often serve as a vital link in transmitting information to the family regarding their relative's condition. They also tend to be physically present in the nursing home more frequently than the physician and, therefore, can perform timely evaluations of any acute medical changes that may have occurred. This often allows any new medical problems to be potentially diagnosed in the facility rather than causing the emotional and physical discomfit of transferring a nursing home resident to an emergency department of a local hospital for such an evaluation. However, not all medical tests can be done within the facility and the physician will decide when it is most appropriate to transport someone to the hospital. Your input on these decisions, however, can be very important. You should get any contact information you can at the time of admission on how to reach the NP or PA if your doctor utilizes the services of such an individual.

Nurses

Each unit at a nursing home has nurses assigned to care for your relative. These may be registered nurses (RNs) or licensed practical nurses (LPNs). Throughout the stay, the nurses are responsible for the total care of your loved one and oversee the day-to-day care routines of the certified nursing assistants (see below). Any questions or concerns with care you may have should first be brought to the attention of the unit nurse assigned to your relative. The day shift nurses usually will have the ability to obtain answers for you in the most timely manner.

Certified Nursing Assistants (CNAs)

The CNAs are usually, but not always, high school graduates who have received at least seventy-five hours of training in the care of the older adult in the nursing home setting. They are almost always the lowest paid employee of the facility and often have a high "turnover" rate, with up to 100 percent of newly hired individuals quitting the job within the first year of employment. Despite these issues, the typical CNA performs in excess of 90 percent of the hands-on care to all of the residents in the nursing home. These duties include grooming, bathing, toileting, dressing, mouth care, ambulation and responding to any call lights that are activated by the resident at any time. All CNAs are supervised by the nurse in charge of that unit.

Most CNAs have approximately ten residents assigned to them on the day shift and this number may increase on evening and night shifts depending on the staffing available on any given shift. The assignments may vary by the care requirements of the residents and the total workload but the assignments are typically divided fairly among the CNAs on duty. As such, they are often very busy. It is very important for you to get to know the CNAs that are assigned to your relative as they can provide a wealth of information on their current condition and any recent changes or issues that may have arisen. It is also very useful if you can tell the various assigned CNAs any special needs, likes, dislikes or other special care requirements so they can provide the best possible care.

At times you may hear many negative comments about CNAs. As Karen Shoff, MSW, has said, "Nursing homes are the McDonalds of the healthcare world—employing a roster of unskilled individuals for the lowest possible wage." Many facilities, though, have a significant number of highly skilled and dedicated CNAs despite the low wages and demanding working conditions. The more you can support and assist the CNA assigned to your relative, the better the care that will be delivered. If you have concerns regarding the care being delivered you should speak to the nurse on duty for that particular unit or the charge nurse on the day shift.

Dentists

Dental care is a critical component of an overall health prevention plan for all nursing home residents. Although fees charged by dentists are not routinely covered by the Medicare program (but are covered under Medicaid) it is still very important that families continue to arrange comprehensive dental care on a regular basis for their relative. Most facilities do not have a dentist that visits on-site as much of the usual treatments require equipment and staff support not readily available at a nursing home. Dental appointments and transportation will have to be arranged and paid for by the family.

Inform the nurse in charge of the unit when a dental appointment is made so that an accurate copy of the current medication list or other requested records for the dentist can be ready on the day of the visit. Twice a year checkups and cleanings should be maintained. Loose fitting dentures need to be evaluated and repaired by the dentist as soon as the problem is noted as poorly fitting dentures can affect nutritional status.

Social Workers

Social workers are available to meet the social and psychological needs of all residents. They may assist you in

- education regarding the nursing home and the different resources available,
- counseling and support services relating to an individual's ability to cope with illness and other chronic problems (e.g., dementia and related diseases),
- referrals to specialists or other support organizations,
- obtaining information on discharge planning, advance directives and resident rights and responsibilities,
- discussing potential room changes,
- facilitating communication of medical information to other agencies,
- giving selected guidance in developing certain aspects of the plan of care for your relative,

- answering basic insurance questions and determining if benefits are available, and
- informing you of various facility activities and programs that are available.

Dietitian

At the time of admission a diet order will be given by the admitting physician. The dietitian will also do a formal evaluation of the nutritional needs of your relative shortly after admission and make any recommendations regarding any special nutritional or fluid needs. These recommendations need to be approved by the physician before they can be put into effect.

If your relative has any special dietary needs or favorite foods (including religious preferences) make sure you contact the dietitian to let them know so they can adjust the diet accordingly. Any allergies to foods should also be noted and inform the nursing staff of these items.

Speech and Audiology

Audiologists and speech pathologists can provide hearing and speech evaluations as well as make treatment recommendations for your relative. Some facilities may have contracts with local audiologists who may arrange on-site visits but, if not, you should feel free to make an appointment with a community-based company after discussing your concerns with the physician. If a new hearing loss is suspected please be sure to speak with the physician first so they may check for any ear wax impaction, as this is a common cause of hearing loss in nursing home residents.

Rehabilitation, Occupational and Physical Therapists

Should your relative need to relearn certain skills, physical and occupational therapists are available to provide such services. This therapy must be ordered by the physician and usually follows a request for a therapy evaluation. These therapists will also assist in teaching your relative how to use certain assistive devices such as walkers, artificial limbs and wheelchairs. The therapists, who usually work on-site within the nursing home, can help to teach an individual how to bathe, dress and eat again if needed. Some of the therapy costs may be covered by Medicare Part A if the nursing home stay is occurring just after an acute hospital stay for a qualifying medical illness (such as stroke, pneumonia with deconditioning or after hip repair surgery). The facility's social worker can assist you with regards to determining if any requested services are covered under Medicare Part A. Therapy costs for some residents may also be covered under Medicare Part B. Therapy is usually limited by the ability to reach certain therapeutic goals and how one responds to the rehabilitative program.

Recreational Therapist

A recreational therapist can provide activities that meet the psychosocial needs of all residents. The therapist typically completes an assessment on all new admissions and may design activities that can meet identified treatment goals and also provide a social atmosphere. Diversional activities are planned and can include games (e.g., bingo), movies, cookouts, trips to local activities and arts and crafts. An activity calendar is always posted that lists the coming day's events. Activities are required to be scheduled seven days a week and family members may often participate in some of the scheduled activities.

Chaplains

Chaplains of various faiths are available to assist in meeting the spiritual needs of the residents. Most of the clergy are available "on call" and the social worker can help to arrange a visit when needed. You may also take your relative out (with the permission of the physician) to attend services at your usual place of worship. Personal visits by your own clergy to the nursing home are also encouraged and welcome.

Chapter 3

Communicating with the Attending Physician: How to Avoid Frustration

You are told by the Dean on day one of medical school that 50 percent of what you will be learning will be obsolete in ten years. "The problem is," he continues, "we don't know *which* fifty percent."
—Old medical school joke

The typical physician (doctor) today is asked to work longer hours, care for more patients and accept less reimbursement for any work he or she does. This does not normally allow doctors to spend substantial amounts of time on the telephone or in person discussing the care of a relative in a nursing home with various family members. Many doctors who care for residents in a nursing home do so in addition to working a full day at their office or many hours in the hospital. As such, doctors often make rounds on their nursing home residents late in the day or early in the evening. As federal regulations only require visits to the nursing home every sixty days (after monthly visits for the first three months following admission), the physical presence of the doctor providing medical care for your loved one may be relatively rare. This does *not* mean that your relative is receiving bad care or that the doctor is unaware of what is happening. The doctor relies on the nursing staff and family members to alert him or her if something does not appear to be going well or if there is a change in the physical or mental condition of one of their residents. Tips for talking with the doctor are given in Table 3.1. At the time of admission, be sure to get the name of the doctor and his or her telephone number as well as that of any nurse practitioner or physician assistant they may work with in the nursing home.

Table 3.1
Tips for Talking with a Physician or Healthcare Provider

- Make a list of the questions you want to ask in order of priority.
- Make an appointment to discuss issues in person or by telephone.
- Keep your comments and questions brief and to the point.
- If you have questions regarding medications, make a list of the medications you wish to discuss.
- If you do not understand the answer you are given, ask for a further explanation right then and there.
- If you have specific care requests, make sure the doctor understands what you desire.
- Talking with the nurse practitioner may also be beneficial in obtaining the most up-to-date information on your loved one.

When you discuss your relative with the doctor (who is also called the **attending physician**), nurse practitioner or physician assistant (which we will refer to in this book as **healthcare providers**), make sure you have your concerns organized and be as concise as possible. Many times the nurse practitioner or physician assistant will be present in the facility on a fairly regular basis and can answer or directly intervene on behalf of the doctor for most clinical concerns you might have. If they have any areas they wish to discuss with the supervising doctor, they can contact him or her directly. The doctor, nurse practitioner or physician's assistant can also assist in arranging consultations with other specialists, such as podiatry, psychiatry, psychology, neurology, cardiology or gastroenterology.

If you have questions about any of the medications that have been prescribed make sure you know which ones you are inquiring about. You may find it useful to make a chart listing all of your relative's medications, the time of day they are being given and the clinical disease or symptom being treated. A sample chart is shown as Table 3.2. If you have concerns regarding any risks associated with any particular medication, ask that question specifically along with requesting if there are alternative medications that could be considered with a lower side effect profile. Common terms that often accompany the instructions for the administration of medications include:

p.r.n. = "as needed"　　　　　a.c. = "before meals"
q.d. = "once every day"　　　p.c. = "after meals"
b.i.d. = "twice a day"　　　　p.o. = "by mouth"
q.i.d. = "four times a day"　　h.s. = "at bedtime"

The vending pharmacist (the individual who works for the pharmacy that delivers all of the medications to the nursing home) is also a good source of information on medications, side effects and potential drug-drug interactions. In addition, they can review the cost of the medicines being dispensed. To make the best use of your time with your loved one's healthcare provider, keep your questions clear and to the point. If you don't understand the answer you are given, do not be afraid to say so and ask for further explanation. The more questions you ask, the more you will learn. Also, do not hesitate to share your point of view with the healthcare provider. Do not forget to review with them any special needs, medication reactions, allergies, habits or other requirements your relative may have at the facility. If you have any other special requests regarding your relative,

Table 3.2
Chart for Medication Use in a Nursing Home

Name of Drug	Dosage	Date Started	How Often	Reason

be sure that the doctor understands the exact nature of what you are seeking. If you find it difficult to reach the healthcare provider ask the administrator or director of nursing of the nursing home to help expedite your inquiries.

It may be useful for you to take notes on what you learn so you can refer to it later if other family members ask you to fill them in on any current issues. It is also helpful to the healthcare provider if the family selects one representative to be the primary contact point or spokesperson for information transfer. This will streamline the process of getting answers to critical questions or requests and help cut down on duplication of efforts.

Always attempt to meet and talk with the other members of healthcare team who will be working with your relative at the facility. These individuals may include the nurses, certified nursing assistants, speech, occupational or physical therapists, dietitians and activity therapist. These professionals may be able to take more time with you and answer some of your questions or concerns more specifically.

Although the Internet has become a valuable tool for obtaining information on a variety of subjects, it is critical for you not to accept everything you read on websites as the absolute truth. Not all information on the Web is of equal quality and this distinction may be difficult to see. Discuss anything you find on the Internet with your healthcare provider so you can hear their opinion.

One of the important areas you should discuss as early as possible with their healthcare provider is that of **advance directives** and **end-of-life planning** for your relative. All nursing homes are required to provide you with information at the time of admission on completing advance directives but it is often not done in great detail due to various time constraints. Advance directives involve developing guidelines regarding the level and type of healthcare interventions for the resident admitted to a nursing home when they can no longer make medical decisions for themselves. A resident of a nursing home who is competent to make medical decisions for him or herself can be asked directly regarding their wishes. This document will assist the facility and furnish the healthcare provider with information on how to approach many care issues, such as the desire for hospitalization, the use of intravenous fluids or medications in times of illness, whether or not to insert a tube for artificial feedings or the potential use of defibrillation and intubation (which involves inserting a tube into the lungs to assist with breathing) in case of cardiac arrest. Only an authorized representative of your relative can sign for a **DNR order**, which means "do not resuscitate" and tells the healthcare facility or provider that if a cardiac or respiratory arrest occurs no interventions will be initiated to reverse nature's course. However, DNR orders do *not* mean that infections or other medical illnesses will not be treated. Examples of authorized representatives may include a spouse, durable power of attorney for healthcare, guardian or other next-of-kin as authorized by state law.

Some individuals may have previously prepared what is called a **living will**, which is a document that outlines the personal wishes regarding life-sustaining treatments by that person. This document can assist the decision-maker and the family in deciding or choosing the level of medical intervention desired if your relative's medical condition deteriorates. (See Appendix E for further information of organizations dealing with end-of-life planning.) Only the legal next-of-kin, guardian or person with power of attorney (**decision-maker**) can actually authorize the level of intervention and each state has laws that specify the details. It is best to have any involved family members meet and decide the limits of intervention before meeting with the healthcare provider. If there are disagreements among the family, the actual legal decision maker will be the one to make the final decision. Remember, even if you decide on one course of treatment or limit certain interventions, these instructions can always be revoked (canceled) at any time by notifying the healthcare provider and the facility of your new wishes.

If you feel the doctor is not being responsive to your needs or does not return your calls in a reasonable time frame (for example, within two days), you may wish to consider switching to another doctor. The nursing home will have a list of available doctors although you may choose any willing and eligible to join the nursing home staff. Asking the staff nurses who the best doctors are (in private, of course) will give you valuable information on selecting a doctor. Since they work with these doctors on a regular basis they will know better than the director of nursing or administrator, who calls back promptly and who appears to show compassion and dedication to providing good, quality nursing home care. Above all, be persistent in keeping the lines of communication open with your doctor.

Chapter 4

Use of Restraints: Physical and Medication-Related

Tying down or medicating someone in a nursing home in order to reduce falls, wandering, elopement risk and agitation leads in time, without fail, to the exact opposite outcome. If we are to civilize our treatment of the older adult, we need to further reduce our dependence on the voodoo magic of restraints.

—Nursing home physician

The continuing use of physical restraints and medications that work in the brain to sedate someone are ongoing issues in nursing homes. Before the enactment of federal legislation in 1987 that severely restricted the acceptable clinical indications for the use of physical and chemical (i.e., drug-induced) restraints in nursing home residents, the routine application of such restraints was fairly commonplace. Restraints, by definition, are any devices or pieces of equipment that cannot be removed by individuals themselves and which causes restriction in their movement. Restraints, by law, can only be applied on the order of a physician and the type of device, indication, authorized time periods for use (including release intervals that are at least every two hours during the day and every four hours during the night) must be specified in the order. Restraints may never be ordered when staffing numbers are low in order to compensate for these shortages or as a punishment initiated by a staff member for perceived "bad behavior" on the part of a resident.

Restraints have many unwanted side effects including decreasing muscle strength, negatively affecting gait, balance and respiratory function and increasing the potential for skin breakdown or the development of limb contractures. Prolonged inactivity from restraints can also lead to decreased bone mineral density (which can weaken the body's bones) and can potentially increase agitation or social withdrawal in residents with dementia. The presence of incontinence can also increase as the ability for a resident to reach a bathroom in a timely manner would be obviously hindered by the use of restraints. Importantly, studies have shown that restraints do *not* decrease the incidence of falls, which is the reason most often given for wanting to use a restraint, or prevent fall-related injuries.

Side rails on beds that do not allow the person to exit on their own are also considered restraints and some types of side rails have been associated with serious injuries and even death. Physical restraints may include any of the following;

- chairs and wheelchairs with lap belts, cushions or trays that prevent egress,
- waist ties,
- mittens,
- wrists ties,
- vests,
- bed rails, and
- Geri Chairs.

Rarely, many of the above types of restraints have led to physical injuries, such as a bone fracture or strangulation and death when not properly used or monitored. All staff members are required to receive inservice training on the proper use of restraints if any of these devices are being used on the unit where they will be assigned to deliver care.

The dignity issue associated with excessive restraint use is also something that can have negative effects on an individual. Being tied down in a restraint can potentially have damaging psychological effects on the individual. The federal government has set strict standards for the use of such devices and if you have any questions regarding their use you should discuss them with the unit charge nurse or the attending physician. Any restraint must be used for an approved clinical indication and it is mandated that the staff release the resident from the device every two hours during the day for ambulation, repositioning, toilet use or other care needs. Often facilities have a **restraint committee** where alternatives to the use of restraints are suggested to address the clinical concern that has prompted consideration for the use of such a device.

A significant number of facilities have attempted to become "restraint-free" and rarely, if ever, allow the use of any of these devices. You may find out the policy at your facility by asking the social worker to obtain for you a copy of the current **restraint policy** in effect. Federal regulations regarding restraint usage may also be obtained by visiting the website for the Centers for Medicare and Medicaid Services at www.cms.gov. Federal regulations regarding "Resident Rights" (see Appendix A) also discuss restraint use.

Medications may also be used that have the effect of "restraining" an individual by sedating them. A medication that is given purely to sedate an individual has typically been referred to as a "chemical restraint," although technically that is not the reason that anyone will routinely admit to as the reason they were ordered. Centrally acting drugs that may cause sedation include the following classes of medications.

- **antipsychotics**. e.g., Zyprexa (olanzapine), Risperdal (risperidone), Seroquel (quetiapine) and Clozaril (clozapine)—known as *atypical* antipsychotics—and others such as Haldol (haloperidol), Mellaril (thioridazine), Thorazine (chlorpromazine) and Stelazine (perphenazine)—known as *conventional* antipsychotics
- **antiseizure**. e.g., Depakote (valproic acid), Tegretol (carbamazepine) and Neurontin (gabapentin)
- **anti-anxiety and tranquilizers**. e.g., Serax (oxazepam), Ativan (lorazepam), Valium (diazepam) and BuSpar (buspirone)

Although antidepressants also work in the brain, they are typically used to treat depression, rather than to sedate an individual. One exception is trazodone (generic name), which is a mild antidepressant often used to aid in inducing sleep.

Federal regulations require that any time an antipsychotic medication is ordered by a physician that a specific target symptom or group of symptoms in a resident be identified and documented as the justification for the use of such a medication. For example, an individual with paranoid thoughts that his food is being poisoned or that hears voices at night would be a legitimate indication for the use of an antipsychotic medication. Although antipsychotics are typically used to treat schizophrenia, many of the hallucinations or paranoid thoughts that are seen in residents with dementia mimic some of the same thought processes seen in schizophrenia and can respond to similar type medications, although in older adults they are usually given in lower dosages. The target symptoms that are being treated are required to be monitored and documented by the staff so the efficacy and any side effects from the medication can be noted. Behaviors such as wandering, yelling, disrobing, urinating in public places or hoarding of items are not usually treated effectively by this class of medications.

All of these classes of medications have potential serious side effects, especially if used in higher doses than recommended for geriatric age groups, and the nursing staff should be knowledgeable about what adverse reactions to look for in any resident receiving such medications. If you notice any change in mental status or functional level of your loved one on such a medication, you should notify the charge nurse immediately so he or she can be evaluated for a potential adverse reaction to the medication.

The next-of-kin should be notified prior to the initiation of any antipsychotic medications and if you have concerns or questions regarding the use of *any* medications, including antipsychotics, insist on having the facility arrange for you to discuss these concerns with the attending physician. All medications that can potentially have an additive effect, and many have drug-drug interactions, can impair an individual's functional ability and mental status. Always review the *entire* list of medications that have been prescribed for your loved one and if you do not understand the reason for the medication being ordered insist on speaking to the nurse practitioner or the attending physician to obtain further clarification or to discuss any potential changes.

Do not hesitate to discuss the continuing need for restraints. For example, if restraints are being used to allow the staff to administer an intravenous medication, once the treatment is over the continued need for the restraint may no longer be present. Additionally, using the least restrictive device or alternatives to restraint use (for example, the use of a Merry Walker instead of a Geri Chair; increased walking activities for restless individuals and so on) is the current standard of care before a restraint can be ordered. Be as active and involved as you can when restraint use is being considered for your loved one and make sure that reevaluation of a continued need for such a device, if ordered, is completed on a regular basis.

Chapter 5

How to Make Visits to Your Loved One Valuable

A visit to a loved one is always more important than one would suspect. It is a bridge to the life and times left behind and maintains the bond to family, friends and especially to memories.

— Nursing home physician

Visiting your loved one in a facility can have many positive aspects including emotional support, assisting in social interaction with other residents, helping with physical movements and can also aid with some care needs if deemed appropriate by the staff. However, it is critical that you develop good communication skills with the staff of the facility to ensure that your loved one receives the best possible care and that your visits will be a rewarding experience for all.

The first step is to read the **resident handbook** (or equivalent title) that is provided to the family free of charge at the time of admission to the facility. This booklet will contain very valuable information about the facility's policies and procedures concerning smoking, storage of valuables, furniture, self-medication, room transfers, visiting, discharges, bedholds and readmission.

When you visit and talk with your loved one, be alert for some of the emotional challenges they may be facing which can include

- separation anxiety from spouse, family and friends from their previous residence,
- a sense of loss of identity when surrounded by large numbers of relative strangers, and
- a loss of independence as the entire day's cycle may now be determined by set schedules, unfamiliar routines and rules.

It is important to help your relative maintain ties with family and community friends as much as possible. Offer to bring over old friends and family members on a regular basis so that these emotional friendships can survive and provide support in the nursing home setting. Encourage your loved one to maintain as much independence as possible within the limits of the facility's policies (e.g., encourage an active role in selecting menu items that are most desired or requesting special activities they may enjoy). Try to realize that more frequent shorter visits are preferable to less frequent longer ones. Sometimes just sitting with an individual and watching a television show together may provide entertainment and emotional support. Table 5.1 lists an effective method of preparing for a quality visit to a nursing home.

If you can provide a VCR and television in your relative's room you can bring their favorite movies in for them to watch. This might be preferable to having to watch whatever program is on the facility's main TV set. Also, you might consider creating your own video of family and friends. For those individuals that can use a telephone calling on a regular basis can almost always improve the individual's spirits.

If you are visiting a loved one with special needs, you may need to make some adjustments in your communication style.

For those residents with hearing impairment:

- Speak more clearly and slower, not louder.
- Keep background noises, music or television volumes at a minimum.
- Repeat words as needed.
- Write down any words on a pad that are not being understood.
- Always maintain good eye contact.
- Watch facial reactions to make sure you are being understood.

For those residents unable to speak or understand well (for example, after a stroke):

- Always give the individual plenty of time to talk.
- Try to ask "yes" or "no" questions as much as possible.
- Write down sentences on a pad.
- Use gestures of face and hands to help convey information.

- Use a message board with the alphabet and a few key words on it (facilities can either provide these for your use or tell you where one can obtain them).

Table 5.1
Tips for Arranging a Quality Visit to a Nursing Home

1. Learn the facility's routines and schedules for meals, group activities and therapy periods. Also, try to determine the best time of day that your relative wishes to receive visitors.
2. Always check with the nursing staff or dietitian before bringing in any food. Make sure food is always sealed in an appropriate container and that it can be safely left at room temperature unless refrigeration has been arranged.
3. Come for your visit with ideas for activities, games, recent photographs or specific conversational topics. Even listening to the radio or watching television together can be important to your loved one.
4. Participate in facility activities when appropriate or work together on a project together such as a puzzle, photo album or other hobby. Place favorite photographs and cards on the room wall as allowed by facility policy.
5. Bring a favorite pet in to visit (when allowed by facility policy).
6. Bring in tape-recorded messages from friends and family who cannot easily visit.
7. Celebrate birthdays and holidays with your relative and family members (plan ahead with facility staff).
8. Bring children and grandchildren to visit whenever possible.
9. Read aloud from hometown newspapers or favorite magazines.
10. Rent books-on-tape on subjects your loved one is interested in hearing (may need to buy inexpensive headsets if tape player to be used at night).
11. Take your loved one out to a local restaurant, a movie or something as simple as ice cream if appropriate and authorized by the attending physician.
12. Videotape or take pictures with your loved one so they can be brought in during your next visit.

For those residents who have visual difficulties or are blind:

- Use words and sentences that paint a colorful picture.
- Bring in books recorded on tape to play with headphones.
- Offer to read magazines or newspapers.
- Bring in a radio tuned to the resident's favorite type of station.
- Purchase a tape player to play preferred music.

Above all, *be patient!* Don't become discouraged to the point where you no longer want to visit if one time events did not go well as you had wished. Remember that short visits more frequently are usually appreciated more by nursing home residents than less frequent but longer visits. Always try to be a good listener and not to finish or interrupt sentences. Show your appreciation to staff members whom are particularly helpful with a sincere word of thanks or a letter of praise to the staff member's supervisor.

If you have concerns regarding the care you see being delivered do not hesitate to speak up, even if it involves another resident in the facility. Table 5.2 lists some suggested ways of voicing these concerns to the nursing home staff. When you communicate care concerns, try not to speak in a threatening manner. Instead, suggest solutions and formulate with the staff a mutually agreeable plan for care concerns.

Overall, visits to your loved one should be a positive experience. Attempt to keep a positive attitude at all times. And, if you fall short during one visit, there is always the next time. As Norman Vincent Peale often said, "Any fact facing us is not as important as our attitude towards it, for that determines our success or failure." Having a loved one in a nursing home *is* a stressful life experience, but one that can be handled if we approach it with understanding, patience, good communication skills and compassion.

Table 5. 2
How to Voice Concerns to the Staff in the Nursing Home

1. Become familiar with the staff members during visits and learn who is in a position and receptive to problem-solve or answering questions. *Do not hesitate to speak up if you see something that bothers you!*
2. Discuss any care concerns with the staff in a nonthreatening manner and try to avoid exhibiting any excessive emotional reaction.
3. Suggest possible solutions to the staff member or arrange for the care team to meet as a group at a mutually convenient time to discuss your concerns.

Chapter 6

How to Monitor Care and Encourage Good Teamwork

It is somehow ironic that, for residents of nursing homes, the individuals- the certified nursing assistants- to whom we assign the bulk of the hands-on care such as feeding, dressing, toileting and walking, routinely get paid the least amount of money. Additionally, learning to take criticism well from visiting family members is a skill few nursing assistants possess and even fewer desire to learn it.

—Nursing home physician

The typical family member almost always has concerns about how well their relative will be treated by complete strangers in a nursing home setting. Monitoring the care they receive is something that many individuals often feel is being done by another entity, such as state inspectors or ombudsman representatives. In truth, routine required inspections (usually done yearly) or a complaint investigation by a state agency or other organization will never replace the important need for family members to monitor the care being given in the facility on a regular basis. Additionally, it is important to keep track of personal items (e.g., radios, electric razors, tape players and VCRs) or medical equipment that may become lost or misplaced in another resident's room by mistake.

One of the most common problems family members will encounter in the nursing home is the loss of their loved one's personal items. Clothing is most commonly misplaced after wearing or in the facility laundry system. Always ensure that all items of clothing, including socks and shoes are labeled with the resident's name written on them with an indelible marker. You should also start and regularly update an inventory list of clothing and personal items and make sure the nursing staff has a copy of this list for the chart. Many nursing homes will complete such an inventory for you at the time of admission.

Dentures and hearing aids, which are important to the resident's quality of life, can also become lost and are quite costly to replace. To help prevent their loss, ask the charge nurse of the unit to instruct the staff to insert the hearing aid each morning and collect it each night so it can be locked or placed in a safe place (e.g., in the medication cart or medication room). This procedure will ensure the nursing staff will be accountable and there will be a record of who handled the personal items last.

Before admission or shortly thereafter, ask your dentist to label any dentures with your relative's name as this needs to be done with a special engraving tool. Wheelchairs, walkers, canes, splints, braces or any other medical equipment should also be labeled with the resident's name.

Other valuable personal items, such as rings, diamonds, necklaces, money, bracelets, watches or similar items should be removed at the time of admission and taken home by the next-of-kin. If your loved one is accustomed to wearing a diamond ring and is upset at the removal of the jewelry, consider purchasing an inexpensive replacement that can be used. Expensive jewelry can become the target of others and additional personal insurance for valuable items should be obtained if these items remain in the facility. Facility insurance policies do *not* cover the loss of any personal items.

Family members should get in the habit of regularly checking for personal items during visits to verify they have not been misplaced. If an item is recognized as missing, a search of the room should be conducted first as many times items are placed in different locations. If it is an item of clothing, the laundry room should also be checked. If it is not found, report it to the licensed nurse in charge of your relative immediately.

Most of the time a thorough search will locate the items. However, if these procedures do not work, the nursing staff should conduct a room-to-room search if the items are costly in nature or important to the resident's health. Trash containers and the dining room area should also be searched. Remember, sometimes an individual with dementia may accidentally place an item in another resident's room, or remove their dentures or hearing aids and leave them in an unusual place. If an item is not found, request the nursing staff to complete an incident report that may be useful if an insurance claim is to be made. The nursing supervisor and director of nursing should also be informed. A written letter to the facility's administrator should be sent identifying in detail the missing items and it is important that you specifically request a reply.

If it is subsequently determined that the nursing home staff were responsible for the loss of the item (e.g., dentures on a food tray that were thrown away), the cost of replacement may be paid by the facility. Any such payment requires the approval of the administrator and this would need to be directly discussed with him or her.

Helping the staff to learn about your loved one is critical to their emotional well-being and the level of care they require. This information should be conveyed to the facility social worker and unit staff and should cover minimally the following areas:

- main reason for nursing home admission,
- children or relatives who are actively involved in your loved one's life,
- all relevant contact information (home and telephone work numbers, cell phones, beepers),
- financial issues,
- name of spouse (if living) or date of divorce or death; current relationship,
- hobbies (discuss with activities coordinator),
- daily habits (naptime, denture or hearing aid routines),
- personal hygiene issues (bathing preference, shaving method and so on),
- favorite tv or radio shows,
- smoking habits (if applicable),
- favorite foods, and
- inclination to receiving affection from staff (hugs or touching).

Concerns may also arise with medical and nursing care within the facility. Any such issues noticed by a family member should be immediately brought to the attention of the licensed nurse in charge. The nurse can then either answer any concerns or intervene with the staff to correct the problem if indicated. Do not hesitate to speak up but attempt to be as non-confrontational as the situation allows. Raising one's voice and threatening are rarely productive in improving care in the long run. If there are any concerns that cannot be resolved at this level, then make an appointment to meet with the director of nursing or the administrator.

The nursing staff is also responsible for notifying the family when there is a change in your relative's mental or physical condition and therefore it is very important that you always leave updated telephone numbers on the chart where you can be reached. If you plan to be out of town, inform the staff of your temporary location and contact information so it can be posted on the chart in the appropriate section. The social worker for the facility can help coordinate the updating of contact information for you.

Medicare Part A nursing home stays ("rehabilitation stays") that follow a three-day qualifying hospital admission may last *up to* 100 days if clinically appropriate, although most stays in these units do not reach the 100 day maximum. Individuals in these units require a higher level of nursing care and specialized services such as physical, occupational or speech therapies. Many of these units can also provide intravenous therapy, specialized wound care and increased monitoring of residents beyond that on the regular floors of the nursing facility. Many of the individuals in this unit may have medical conditions or illnesses that can quickly become unstable. If you notice a change in your loved one's condition while they are in this unit, it is very important that the nursing staff know of your concern right away. If it seems serious, insist that the attending physician be contacted. The quicker a medical problem is addressed, the earlier an effective evaluation or treatment can be ordered and implemented.

Remember, many medical conditions can decline as an underlying disease process progresses. For medical conditions such as stroke and dementia, declines can be expected to occur over the course of years. This progression of the disease can lead to functional and mental declines and would be considered a "natural" progression of an existing condition.

Case Study

Ms. Smith was admitted to Sky View Nursing Facility in January of 2001 with a primary diagnosis of moderate dementia. At the time of admission she was able to walk without assistance, feed and dress herself and could communicate fairly well but had evidence of moderate memory loss. By January of 2003 she now required assistance with feeding, dressing and ambulation and her words could no longer could be clearly understood.

Her physician attributed Ms. Smith's decline to a natural progression of her underlying disease.

Additionally, acute illnesses occurring concurrently in a resident with dementia can have bad outcomes if not treated aggressively in a timely manner. For example, a resident with dementia comes down with pneumonia or a bladder infection associated with a low-grade fever. An examination may reveal a change in functional abilities or mental status. An individual with dementia and an underlying infection may appear more confused, agitated and become uncooperative. This condition is called an acute **delirium**. Unless the underlying infection is treated properly, this condition may progress and lead to a generalized dissemination of the bacteria into the blood stream which is called **sepsis**. Antibiotics and intravenous fluids are required to treat bacterial infections and many individuals will require hospitalization. Mental status and functional ability should return to baseline if the illness has been treated in a timely manner.

In terms of facility-wide monitoring of your loved one's progress, there are **care plan meetings** held approximately every three months that review the overall treatment plan and other issues regarding each resident in the facility. It is critical that a family member attend these meetings if at all possible. Present at these meetings will be representatives of many different departments, including social service, activities, dietary and nursing. Any care concerns can be addressed at this meeting and alterations to the treatment plan made as appropriate. The use of restraints or sedating types of medications is also discussed at these meetings. If medical issues arise, these will be referred to the attending physician for follow-up as needed. If a family member cannot make the scheduled time, ask that the time be altered to fit your schedule as you have a right to be at this meeting to review each department's current assessment and plan for your loved one. You will be notified of the date for the next care plan meeting in advance so you will be able to check your schedule.

Additionally, every attempt should be made for a family member to attend scheduled **resident or family council meetings**. These are facility-wide meetings, usually held monthly or quarterly, where residents and their families can meet and discuss care and facility-related issues. Attending these sessions will give you a chance to see what concerns or issues other family members have identified. Do not hesitate to share your experiences with family members. Also, feel free to talk with state survey-ors when they are making their annual inspection of the building.

There are times when roommates will not get along well. If your rela-tive does not have a private room (which is a higher monthly rate), and you notice that the assigned roommate is not getting along well with your loved one, discuss a possible room change with the social worker. Also, any room changes being contemplated by the staff for your relative must be preceded by family notification. If you are unhappy with the proposed room change, notify the social worker officially prior to the move date and discuss the issue with her. If you are not satisfied with the outcome of this meeting, make an appointment to discuss your concerns regarding such a move with the administrator. Frequent moves can be very disorienting to a resident with dementia and should be kept to a minimum if at all possible.

Monitoring care often requires families to look for "red flags" that may indicate a problem is present. While many of these issues can be eas-ily addressed, an ongoing pattern of repeat lapses may indicate there are system-wide problems in the facility that will require further investiga-tion. A checklist of potential care issues follows (see also Appendix D). Ensuring that the staff assist your relative to the bathroom as often as re-quired (for those residents who cannot ambulate independently) is critical to help avoid the development of incontinence. If staff tell you they are "too busy" to help your relative to the bathroom as required, this needs to be reported up the chain of command. The overall philosophy of the facil-ity should be to encourage the maintenance of as much independence on the part of the resident in dressing, eating, walking, transferring and bath-ing as the underlying medical condition allows. If a restraint has been or-dered for your loved one (see Chapter 4), it is important to make sure the device is being released at least every two hours as required to allow for turning, repositioning and toileting. If you have questions regarding re-straints, discuss these with the unit charge nurse or the attending physi-cian.

Check for the following "red flags" during facility visits

- missing or nonworking hearing aids
- missing or broken eyeglasses

- missing, dirty or broken dentures
- evidence of lack of personal grooming or dirty clothing
- development of new bowel or bladder incontinence that has not been evaluated
- poor foot and nail care
- evidence of meals being served cold, late or not eaten
- decreased oral fluid intake
- development of skin breakdown over the back or heels (pressure ulcers)
- change in functional status or overall mental status that has occurred over a short period of time and has not been evaluated
- onset of new fevers that have not been evaluated
- observed roughness or rudeness by the staff to any residents of the facility
- observed lack of privacy being given to the residents during care period (for example, failing to knock on doors before entering, not drawing curtains around bed and so on)
- observed long delays (more than five minutes) in having call light answered
- lack of organized and meaningful activities seven days a week
- smells or evidence of poor sanitary conditions
- trash containers that are not emptied regularly
- multiple medication errors over the course of several weeks (wrong medication being given)
- toilet procedures are not being carried out as ordered
- restraints are not being released at least every two hours

Working with nursing staff and other allied health providers in a cooperative and team-like manner is the best way to monitor care and obtain prompt and effective interventions when you notice a care issue that needs to be addressed. Most issues can be resolved to your satisfaction if you are persistent and clear in what you are unhappy with. You should make an effort to become familiar with all of the assigned certified nursing assistants (CNAs) and tell them about any of your relative's special habits, likes and dislikes that will assist them in caring for him or her.

Making visits at different times of the day and on different days of the week will also give you a better picture of the care being given to your relative and may help identify lapses in care that may need to be addressed with the facility staff or administration. If you have attempted to resolve any concerns with the CNAs and licensed nursing staff and are still unhappy, a discussion with the director of nursing, the administrator or both would be the next step. They have the ultimate responsibility for everything that goes on in the nursing home. Unresolved medical issues or medication questions should be directed to the attending physician for discussion.

Many families and residents fear that if they complain about care issues that the staff will retaliate against them. For example, some may feel that complaining about the time it takes a staff member to answer a call light may result in resentment toward their loved one and an even greater lack of care when you are not around to see what is happening. However, being assertive in protecting your relative's rights and well-being is almost always in your and their best interests. However, try to focus on those areas that truly are most important to maintaining the highest quality of life for your relative. For example, complaining that there is dust under the bed may not be as important as ensuring that meals are served on time, are hot and taste good. Before accusing any of the staff of not doing their job, explain your concerns clearly and listen to their explanation. Then, decide on a mutually agreeable solution. Also, monitor the tone of your voice as people often react more to the tone of your voice than the actual words. If your tone is angry or nasty in nature, you may not get the cooperation needed to address problems you have identified. *Always* talk with a positive tone in your voice. Reasonable requests and concerns that you may voice are almost always treated with understanding. Always follow-up at a later date to make sure the issue has been properly addressed. Remember to thank staff for work well done. Although tipping is not permitted, buying a basket of fruit or a box of candy for the unit staff to enjoy is always appreciated.

The ombudsman program for long-term care is available in all fifty states and serves to help individuals and families resolves care issues. Each facility must post the name and contact information for the local ombudsman representative. These individuals are either paid or volunteers who have received special training to serve as advocates for the individual residents and their families. They are not mediators but primarily function as a representative of the resident. They are empowered to conduct their own investigations into care and related issues in the facility and can prove an invaluable source of help to the family when other methods have failed to adequately address the issues that have been raised. The outcome of their efforts will depend on the willingness of the facility administration to work cooperatively with them. There is no cost to you to use the ombudsman program. A list of the state contact numbers for ombudsman programs can be found in Appendix B.

Serious allegations that are substantiated by the ombudsman can be referred to the state survey and inspection agencies with the permission of the resident (or the legal next-of-kin when the resident cannot give consent). Families also have the right to file formal complaints with the office charged with licensing and overseeing the nursing facilities in the state. Telephone numbers for these agencies can be found in the "Government Listings" section of your telephone directory. Remember, however, with over 17,000 nursing homes in this country, ombudsmen cannot replace the vital role families play in the monitoring of care for their loved one.

In the end, if all attempts to resolve specific concerns fail, you may wish to consider transferring your loved one to another facility. Although this involves a great deal of paperwork, inconvenience and possible confusion to a resident with dementia, it may be the only way to resolve certain care concerns. Some family members seem to want to continue to yell or "have an attitude" with staff rather than consider transfer to another location, but confrontational methods rarely improve care. Always try to discuss your concerns when you have them and do not become frustrated if you need to repeat the same instructions more than once to the same staff member. Monitoring care is an ongoing process and requires patience, vigilance and good emotional control. Overall, visiting as often as possible remains the best method of ensuring good care and providing emotional support for the resident.

A flow chart summarizing a recommended approach for resolving care concerns follows. Remember that follow-up by the family on a regular basis for any identified clinical issue is critical to ensure that things have been resolved. With a little extra effort and a true desire to "do good" for the resident, the whole nursing home stay can be a positive experience by which everyone comes out ahead.

Recommended Flow Chart for Resolving Clinical Care Concerns in a Nursing Home

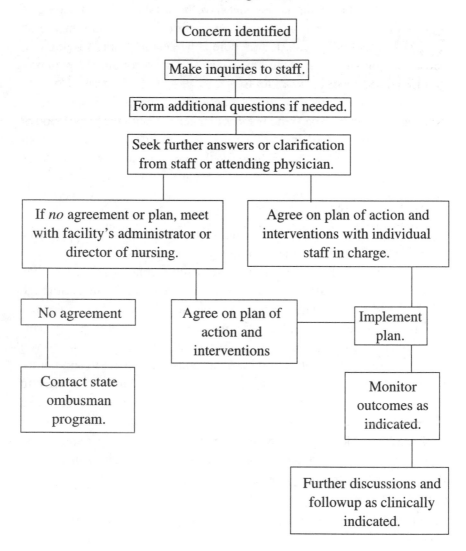

Chapter 7

Can an Attorney Ever Help? Guidelines and Expectations

The first thing we do, let's kill all the lawyers.

—*Henry VI,* Shakespeare

Nursing home litigation has grown to epidemic proportions in the last decade, especially in the south and west. Although rare, you can occasionally read in newspapers of jury verdicts against nursing homes ranging into the tens of millions of dollars. Many law firms nowadays typically advertise on radio, television or in the yellow pages of their expertise in handling litigation against a nursing home. A typical ad might read as follows:

Have you had a loved one who was neglected or injured at a nursing home? Contact us for a free consultation to protect your rights. There is no cost to you if we don't collect. Call us now at . . . .

It may take as long as three years for a case, once filed, to actually reach a courtroom. However, as many as 90 percent of lawsuits settle *before* an actual trial is held, usually just before the trial date is reached. Before the trial, there may be years of discovery (collecting evidence), depositions and mediations. Because of the extended time period between the filing of the lawsuit and any eventual resolution, the original plaintiff (the nursing home resident) may no longer be alive and a child would have to file the action on behalf of the estate.

Filing a lawsuit, while it may be quite appropriate when poor care was given at a nursing home or tolerated by the administration, does not improve any concerns or issues you have *right now*. It is *not* a mechanism to achieve better care for your loved one at the time it is most needed. Some families often develop a sense that their loved one received "bad" care at a

45

facility and then will seek out an attorney in order to obtain monetary compensation and to "send a message" to the nursing home's administrator so the nursing home staff will not let the same incident occur to others in the future.

In general, most nursing homes carry insurance to cover such lawsuits and immediately refer such matters to the attorneys that are hired by the insurance company. The effect of lawsuits on "improving care" is debatable as many of the settlements are associated with a "gag" rule that prevents any discussion of the clinical care issues with the facility staff. Thus, any teaching points that could be made from mistakes is rarely allowed to be disseminated to those who would benefit from it most.

Rarely a family will file a lawsuit while their loved one is still a resident at a nursing home. While some think this may lead to retaliation or the delivery of poor care to the resident, the opposite is probably more likely to occur. However, one would find communication with the staff and administration much more strained and unhelpful as to avoid saying anything that may later be used in a courtroom. Overall, lawsuits probably are the least effective way to improve care for your relative and will definitely set up an adversarial relationship with everyone.

The four criteria that must be satisfied in order for a malpractice action to have merit include:

1. Did the named individual or institution have an established duty or obligation to perform a particular service, provide care to an individual or both?
2. Was there a breach of this duty that fell below the applicable standard of care?
3. Was there an injury to the individual that occurred?
4. Was there a proximate cause that links the breach of duty directly to the injury being alleged by the plaintiff?

If you have decided to seek legal advice, check the local yellow pages for those attorneys who appear to specialize in nursing home-related litigation. Initial consultations should be at no cost to you. If the law firm believes you may have an actionable case, the usual arrangement (which *can vary* from firm to firm) is to agree to receive compensation of 33 percent of any money received plus the costs of handling the lawsuit. It may cost up to $50,000 or more to bring a case to actual trial, so "small" settle-ment amounts may end up giving the family very insignificant compensa-tion when the third of the money is added to the firm's carrying costs of the lawsuit. Some firms may charge the family for getting the nursing home records reviewed by an outside expert, which may cost several thou-sands of dollars depending on the number of pages to be read. Most ex-perts charge between $150 and $450 per hour to read and review records and related documents. Rather than pay for records review, research the various law firms in your area and select one that does not charge you for the initial review. A telephone inquiry can help you determine each par-ticular firm's policies and fees. Remember, there may be years of waiting time until your case is heard and families need to have extreme patience.

Often, just before trial, a settlement offer may be made by the insur-ance company. If you believe the settlement is just, it is useful to consider accepting it and avoid the stress and uncertain outcome of a trial. That decision should be made after discussing the matter with your attorney. Remember, if you lose at trial you will receive no compensation at all.

Having said all this, avoiding the use of attorneys and working in a team-like manner with the staff and administration of a nursing home to improve care is probably the best method of addressing any unresolved concerns. The use of lawsuits is best reserved for gross negligence and deviation from the standard of care on the part of the nursing home admin-istration and staff.

Chapter 8

Final Thoughts

Children often face the difficult prospect of becoming parents to their own parents when dementia or severe medical illness strikes. These children often are in the situation of parenting to their own children at the same time. We must always strive to understand that caring for a family member is rarely easy, often involves significant travel and time commitments and is *never* financially profitable. However, the satisfaction of meeting this challenge well is clearly its own most valuable reward for us. This satisfaction will help us through the void when our loved one is gone and only alive in the echoes of our memories and the tattered photographs that remain behind. We need to teach our own children the importance of family and the love that accompanies the passing of this commitment from one generation to the next.

—Grandson of an Alzheimer's patient

Nursing home placement can be a stressful and emotionally traumatic event for anyone faced with that responsibility. However, the real task that confronts the family begins *after* placement and involves the oversight of the day-to-day care of the individual in the nursing home. This task can literally consume many hours each week of the family's time.

Good communication between the family and the staff at the nursing home can help make this arduous task much easier. However, you may find that consistent good communication on a consistent basis is often lacking and staff may rotate assignments, be occasionally overworked or extremely busy and these events can often lead to frustration for everyone involved. Do not despair. If you keep your goals clear and you stay committed to following-up on clinical and social issues as they arise you will find the stress of overseeing the care at a nursing home can be better tolerated.

Not all accidents in nursing homes can be prevented and the level of care you personally observe can vary from hour to hour or shift to shift within any given nursing home. This does not mean they are providing "bad" care to your loved one. It just means that there are always risks of injury or variations in care patterns that are not easily addressed every hour of the day. The overall goal of this book was to give you the knowledge or the tools needed to assess the ongoing care and to maximize your ability to talk to the staff and attending physician in order to make sure you understand exactly what is happening to your loved one.

Although in recent years there has been an epidemic of attorneys suing nursing homes, lawsuits will not specifically improve the care of your loved one. As they may take up to three or more years to reach a courtroom, it is imperative that you be involved in any care issues immediately. You should understand that if an unexpected accident or injury occurs, this does not "automatically" indicate that neglect or abuse has occurred. The only way to determine culpability or liability for a situation is to gather the facts surrounding the event. Is someone or the facility responsible by not providing the standard of care or adequate supervision of a resident, therefore allowing the accident to happen or is it simply an unforeseen and unavoidable accident or mishap?

Review the "Fifty Most Commonly Asked Questions" in Chapter 9 in order to better understand some of the common issues that may arise from day-to-day in any nursing home. Also, never be afraid to question anything that does not make sense to you, but remember to be as courteous in your inquiries as possible. Staff members tend to respond better to straightforward questions rather than emotionally-laden outbursts from family members directed at anyone in earshot.

With over 1.7 million residents living in nursing homes at the current time (in 2003) the ability to provide quality care to all remains an ongoing challenge. Do not hesitate to contact your state senator and representative to request they commit themselves to improving long-term care in your state and ask them to speak out on this issue during their campaign for re-election. Many states "underfund" Medicaid reimbursement for nursing home beds, which can lead to lower staffing levels. Remember, it is the state representatives and senators, not the federal Senate and House of Representatives, who control the Medicaid rate schedule for their own individual state. The more families help to educate our state representatives and senators regarding the need for improved funding and staffing of our nursing homes, the more advantaged each state's long-term care program will hopefully become.

If there are Alzheimer's support groups in your area, join them to further your understanding of the disease and enhance your coping skills in dealing with memory loss and behavioral changes. These things happen by speaking with others caring for a relative with Alzheimer's disease who are going through much of the same things that you are. Learn from their experiences and share yours with them. Talking and sharing with others is a process that strengthens your inner being and gives you the ability to cope with the routine events or trials of the next day. Volunteering at the nursing home may also give you a better appreciation of the difficulties and challenges the nursing home industry faces daily and perhaps alter any initial misperceptions you might have held regarding the facility.

Do not neglect your own life. Many of us have significant others, children and careers that can occupy any free moments we might occasionally have but it is important to always leave sometime for yourself. Think of your car engine being driven at 120 mph down an empty road. Yes, the engine will carry you but eventually will burn out from the excessive speed and mechanical failure. Never let your own body "burn out" by driving it relentlessly through the traffic of everyday life. Keep up your hobbies, exercise, go to a movie, read a good book and take vacations on a regular basis. These critical breaks from the whirlwind activities we commit ourselves to permit us to regroup our thoughts and perspective, our inner strength and have renewed energy and vitality for life. Don't ever lose your sense of humor.

Above all, keep up your spirits! There are always people you can speak with to relieve some of the stress and guilt you may harbor inside. Keeping your sense of humor will also help, even during periods of high anxiety. Keep this book handy in case questions arise and don't ever give up!

Chapter 9

Fifty Most Commonly Asked Questions about Nursing Homes

1. Is it ever proper to tip employees of a nursing home or give them gifts?

It is never proper to give tips to nursing home staff for services provided to your loved one. However, often at holiday time a gift that can be shared by all employees on that wing (e.g., fruit basket, candy or box of chocolates) is certainly acceptable and usually much appreciated by the staff. If you feel intent on providing a monetary show of your appreciation for the care given, consider donating to the resident fund of the nursing home or the activity department so that the money can be used to help the residents with future projects or trips.

2. How many nursing homes should I visit before deciding on placement?

After discussing what level of nursing home care would be appropriate with your loved one's physician or the hospital staff, make a list of the nursing homes in your area that would meet these needs. If subacute care is required, ask the social worker at the hospital to give you the names of those facilities that offer this specialized level of care. Local churches or synagogues may also offer suggestions if you are looking for a nursing home with a more religious atmosphere. Do not forget to consider location to you and your family as one of the factors.

3. Should the quality of the nursing home be a more important factor than the closeness to relatives?

There is no easy answer to this question. Visits from family members are very important and placing a loved one in a nursing home where the family finds it difficult to frequently visit can have a devastating effect on the overall health and happiness of your relative and can cause guilty feelings to rise up in your mind. Try to arrive at the best compromise possible.

4.   If my parent is living in another state, can I arrange admission to a local nursing home in my own community?
You certainly can. However, you should consider any attachments to new friends or staff that may have been made by your relative during the time they have spent in their current living arrangement. You will also find that it may involve considerable paperwork and time. You will need to:

   a. Find a nursing home with an available bed.
   b. Notify the current nursing home of your intentions to move your loved one at least thirty days in advance so that all needed documents for the new nursing home can be prepared.
   c. You must find a doctor willing to assume medical care immediately upon transfer. Typically the accepting nursing home will have a list of doctors that attend at their facility and can refer you to them. He or she will most likely request that you personally arrange for your relative's medical records to be sent before transfer. This will allow the doctor to become familiar with any special medical needs or treatments and help facilitate continuity of care.
   d. Contact the current attending doctor at the nursing home and notify him of your intention to transfer your loved one to another state. You must ask him to write a transfer order. Do not expect the nursing home to contact him.
   e. You must arrange all necessary transportation. Routine transfers of residents between nursing homes is usually not covered by Medicare or other insurance plans. Feel free to discuss modes of available transportation with the attending doctor, social worker or director of nursing.

5.   Can my parents share a room together?
Although it is rare for both a husband and wife to be admitted at the same time, it would be logical to have them share a room assuming that is the desired arrangement they favor. Unfortunately, most nursing homes are not set up to allow male and female occupants to share the same room as

many units share a common bathroom with another two-bed unit. Most nursing homes have a policy prohibiting the sharing of bathrooms by members of the opposite sex. If you are interested in this option, ask the facility's social worker early on in the application process whether this is possible. All nursing home residents have the right to share a room with their spouse if spacing and policies permit this.

6. How much do nursing homes cost?

Nursing homes that provide custodial, twenty-four-hours-a-day care (non-subacute beds) have costs that vary from state to state and can range from $3,000 to over $7,000 per month, depending on a number of factors including the age of the building, whether a private room is selected and other specialized care needs. This rate excludes physician fees, x-rays, physical therapy, medications and laboratory testing, which may, however, be covered by Medicare and other insurance plans. Some individuals do own nursing home insurance policies that pay for room and board but their coverage limits vary greatly and you will need to review the details of coverage if your relative has such a policy.

7. Will Medicare pay for much of the costs?

Medicare will only pay for those stays that qualify for Medicare Part A coverage. Some of the specific eligibility requirements are that

a. the individual must have spent three consecutive days in an acute care hospital;
b. the nursing home must have a skilled unit (subacute) and be certified to participate in the Medicare program;
c. the nursing home subacute admission must occur either immediately after discharge from the hospital or within thirty days; and
d. the individual needs skilled nursing care or special rehabilitative services.

The doctor must also verify in writing that the nursing home admission is medically necessary and that the patient requires skilled nursing care or rehabilitative care. As benefits are limited to 100 calendar days per year, it is possible to exhaust the benefits prior to having completed the required treatments. At that time you will either have to pay privately, have another insurance plan cover the remaining stay or arrange for a transfer to a lower level of care.

The Medicare Part A benefit covers all services provided (with the exception of physician visits in the nursing home which are covered by Medicare Part B) for the first twenty days. From the twenty-first to the 100th day, the resident will pay a daily deductible (set every year by the federal government but is usually 20 percent of the daily rate). Some insurance plans will cover this deductible but it is best to check the policy carefully before making such an assumption.

8. What if we can't pay the nursing home bills?
Most facilities will not admit a resident without a payment source. Once all private sources of payment are exhausted, you may apply for Medicaid. Medicaid is a state assistance program designated for people of all ages who cannot afford medical care and meet certain income requirements. Applicants must eventually spend down all of their assets, including most property, in order to receive Medicaid coverage. Each state designs its own financial requirements for eligibility but once a Medicaid number is issued, the state will pay for all nursing home charges including all prescription medications. Also, each state has certain restrictions on the transfer of any assets from a nursing home resident to a relative within three years of applying for a Medicaid number (time varies by state). If you have any questions regarding property or monetary transfers, consult an attorney skilled in estate planning prior to filing for state Medicaid coverage.

9. If my parent's private money runs out, can she be transferred out?
If your relative qualifies for Medicaid, many homes will allow your relative to stay. Check each home's payment and transfer policy before placement.

10. Most nursing homes have a specific pharmacy they use when ordering all their medications. Is it possible to use a different one if I find one that has lower-priced medications?
Often the facility will try to discourage you from changing pharmacies because they would rather deal with only one. Their decision to use a par-

ticular pharmacy is based on a number of different factors. If your relative is on Medicaid, all pharmacy bills are covered by this program and you will have limited rights as to pharmacy choice.

However, if the resident is responsible for paying for their medications, you almost always will have a choice of which pharmacy you prefer to use, so check the prices of the "house" pharmacy with a couple of others in the area. Some families have saved considerable money by shopping around. Please note that just because a pharmacy may charge less, it is also important to determine if they will deliver medications on a seven-day schedule. If they refuse to provide delivery on a daily basis or during the evening in an emergency, they will not be allowed to be the pharmacy of record for your relative. Also, they must agree to provide the medications in the correct packaging system that is being used at the nursing home. Check with the director of nursing prior to admission if this issue is of concern to you.

11. What does Medicare assignment mean?

This refers to Medicare Part B coverage which pays the doctor. Accepting "assignment" means the doctor will allow the federal government to set his or her fee. As an example, if the doctor's usual, customary and reasonable fee for a particular procedure is $100. Medicare may reduce that fee per their schedule to approximately $80 and then pay the doctor 80 percent of that amount ($64). The resident or supplemental insurance company would then pay the doctor the remaining 20 percent ($16) which is the difference between the $80 and the $64. Some states mandate that doctors accept assignment from the Medicare program and the nursing home social worker can help you find out that information.

The resident is also responsible for any annual deductible (which may change yearly) and any non-Medicare covered charges (e.g., personal hygiene items, medications and routine transportation charges for clinic visits).

12. How are the resident's personal funds managed by the facility?

The nursing homes social worker can explain their policy on handling resident monies. Most nursing homes have strict rules and bookkeeping procedures to safeguard funds. The orientation materials given to the family on admission should review the current policy on money issues. Federal regulations also exist that cover resident rights with regards to personal fund management (see Appendix A).

13. Are medications and doctor's fees included in the monthly room charge?

In the vast majority of homes, pharmacy, laboratory, x-ray, physical therapy, speech therapy and doctor fees are the responsibility of the resident unless the individual is on Medicaid. However, many insurance plans, including Medicare, may cover all or part of these fees (with the exception of annual deductibles, co-payments and noncovered services). You should check with your insurance carrier to determine the extent of coverage. If your relative is not currently registered for Medicare and is sixty-five or older, you should ensure that they enroll in this federal program. The social worker can assist you with this process.

14. Are dentistry or dentures covered by Medicare?

Medicare and most medical insurance plans do not cover routine dental exams, fillings, dentures, crowns or root canals, although Medicaid will cover such services (note: not all dentists will accept Medicaid payment for their services because the set fees paid by the state are very low). Medicaid may also limit the type and number of dental procedures authorized or the time interval between these procedures. As a result, improving dental care in nursing homes is an important future priority.

If your relative has a dental insurance plan, some of these items will be paid for up to the plan's limits. As good dental care is critical to maintaining good nutritional health and preventing mouth infections, private payment of required and routine dental work is always a good investment on the family's part.

15. Who is responsible for doing the resident's laundry?

Most nursing homes have laundry facilities on-site and can provide this service to your relative for an additional charge every month. However, you can decline this service and provide clean laundry for your relative yourself. Residents on state Medicaid will have it done for them as part of the usual daily charge paid for by the state. You will be informed regarding the nursing home's laundry policy at the time of admission.

16. What is the best way to choose a doctor?

Ask the nursing staff. They will tell you who they feel are the best doctors working at that nursing home. They interact with these doctors on a regular basis and can often judge those qualities that improve the overall delivery of care to a resident of the facility. Do not feel compelled to take the nursing home's medical director or other "house doctor" if you feel you would like another doctor for your relative. You should base your decision on either your own personal review of the doctors on staff, the recommendations of the nursing staff or by talking directly with different doctors who work at that particular facility. Your relative's own doctor can continue to serve as the attending physician at the facility if they agree to follow the nursing home's policies and meet any other required regulations or requirements. In reality, most community-based doctors do not follow their patients once they are admitted to a local nursing home and you will need to select another doctor at the time of admission.

17. What is a medical director?

The medical director is the doctor who works for the nursing home for a set number of hours each month and assists them with meeting all of the administrative items required by state and federal law. He or she may also serve as the doctor for residents living at the facility. Medical directors often serve on a number of nursing home committees, including the Medical Board, Infection Control Committee, Utilization Review and Restraint Committee. The medical director may also be involved with providing employee physicals and overseeing investigations or other projects within the building.

18. Can my parent change doctors?

You can change your relative's doctor at an time by finding one to assume medical responsibility and making sure he or she meets all current regulations regarding joining the nursing home's staff. (The facility's social worker can help to coordinate the switch.) You need not talk with the current doctor directly, writing a letter or leaving a message with his nurse (not his answering service) is acceptable. Make sure the new doctor knows he or she will be required to visit the home to make the necessary resident visits (usually at least once every sixty days). Again, required doctor visits must be made at the facility and the orders renewed at that time.

19. Can I bring other doctors into a facility to do a consult on my relative?

With the permission of the facility and the current nursing home doctor, you can arrange consultations with other doctors either in the facility or at the doctor's private office. You will be responsible for setting up the appointment time, any required transportation and arranging for the copying of any required medical records for the consulting doctor. Discuss this with the unit charge nurse prior to setting a consultation date. If the doctor will be coming to the facility, he or she will most likely need to have their credentials verified first by the nursing home before they can visit you relative.

20. Do most doctors use nurse practitioners in the nursing homes?

Many, but certainly not all, doctors may use nurse practitioners or physician assistants in their nursing home practices. You should find out the contact information for these individuals if you are told at the time of admission that a nurse practitioner or physician assistant will be working with the doctor in the care of your relative.

21. Where can I get a list of doctors who will go to a particular nursing home?

The facility will give you a list of all doctors who belong to the staff and currently accept new residents. You may also check with your own community doctor regarding any doctors he or she may know that go to nursing homes in the area and whom they can recommended as providing good care. Local hospitals with geriatric sections may also be able to provide a list of doctors that are willing to care for nursing home residents.

22. Is it important that I visit my relative on a regular basis?

All visits are well worth the time (see Chapter 5). Short, more frequent visits are more important than longer, less frequent ones. Encourage friends, neighbors and other relatives to visit on a regular basis. These visits help your relative to maintain important community contacts, feel important to others and keep their spirits up.

23. Will I be notified of any change in my parent's condition?
Yes. By law, nursing homes are required to notify you of any changes in your relative's condition, including falls and minor injuries (assuming that you are the spouse or legal next-of-kin). If you go on vacation or a business trip, always leave a telephone number where you can be reached in an emergency or designate an alternate individual to serve as the contact person while you are away.

24. Can I take my parent home for holidays or weekends?
Yes. Most nursing homes allow home visits or community outings with the permission of the doctor. Some states limit the number of days a resident may stay overnight if they are receiving state Medicaid funding for their stay. Always check with the facility's social worker regarding the current policy.

25. Can the doctor stop me from taking my parent out for visits?
Yes, if the doctor feels such visits would jeopardize the health of your relative or if ordered treatments could not be given while the resident was out of the facility. If you have questions, contact the doctor directly. Sometimes arrangements can be made for the family to administer required medications or treatments with minimal training.

26. Can younger children or pets visit in a nursing home?
Children and even babies are almost always welcome in nursing homes during regular visiting hours. Check with the nursing home for their policy regarding visitation by children and the specific hours the nursing home allows guests. Some homes may prohibit animals or certain types of pets from visiting, but many others either encourage it or will allow it in specific areas of the building. It is best to ask the facility's social worker before attempting to bring any pets into the facility.

27. Are there health hazards to children visiting?
Call the nurse in charge of the unit if you have any concerns regarding visits with a child if your relative is ill. In general, it is not a good idea for anyone who is ill to visit relatives in a nursing home.

28. How often will a doctor see my relative in the nursing home?
Although regulations vary from state to state, it is customary for a doctor to visit the resident in a nursing home at least once every thirty to sixty days, even if they were visited daily in the acute care hospital. Also, a nurse practitioner or physician assistant may be visiting every thirty to sixty days. Importantly, a healthcare provider will always be able to see a resident in an emergency or arrange for transfer to the hospital if more intensive evaluation is needed. In addition, a covering doctor is always available if the primary physician is away for one reason or another.

29. What if they need to be seen more often than the allowed thirty- or sixty-day visits?
If you privately pay the doctor you may request that he or she visit your relative more often than the scheduled thirty or sixty day visits. If you are unhappy with the frequency of the doctor's visits, call and discuss it with him or her. Medicare reimbursement rules sometimes make it more difficult for the doctor to be paid for more than two visits in any thirty-day period in the nursing home. However, if there is a real medical need the person can be seen by the doctor either at the nursing home or at the hospital.

30. If my parent needs daily physical or occupational therapy, is that provided at the nursing home?
Usually only skilled nursing facilities or subacute units provide daily physical, occupational or speech therapy. A doctor's order is needed for these specialty referrals and treatments and the associated fee is separate from the room and board charge (outside of the subacute unit; see Question #7). However, Medicare Part B may cover some of these special services, up to the yearly reimbursement limits set by the federal government, if they are ordered by the doctor. Discuss these issues with the doctor before requesting any therapy treatments.

31. Are activities provided for residents of nursing homes?
Nursing homes are required to provide meaningful activities for all of the residents seven days a week. Most nursing homes have a recreational supervisor whom you can contact for the list of scheduled activities to help determine those that may be of interest to your loved one. Also, be

sure to relay any specific activities your relative may enjoy to the recreation department's staff.

32. If, for some reason, I decide I want a private nurse or aide (part-time) for my parent in a nursing home, is this possible?
Most nursing homes will not object if you hire a private duty nurse or aide, but you must check with the director of nursing prior to doing so. The facility and state will have a list of specific licensing and background checks that must be completed before that individual can work in the building. Regardless of how much you feel this extra help is needed, do not expect Medicare, Medicaid, the facility or other insurance plans to pay for such assistance.

Many facilities will have a list of private duty individuals that have worked there before that you may contact or you can look in the yellow pages of the telephone book under "Nurses" or "Nurse Registries." Do not expect this help to be inexpensive. You may pay well over $20 an hour for aides and over $40 an hour for licensed nurses. You may wish to discuss this issue with the doctor before deciding to hire any private duty help.

33. Do I have a right to know the medications my parent is taking?
If you are the spouse or legal next-of-kin (and your relative is deemed unable to handle his or her own affairs), then you have every right to know the medications. It is important to point out that under new federal legislation that went into effect in 2003, all residents of any healthcare facility have the right to bar disclosure of medical information to any family member if they choose to do so. However, if you are legally entitled to make healthcare decisions for your relative, feel free to talk with the unit charge nurse, the doctor or other healthcare provider regarding any medications being given.

34. What do I do if my relative is being bothered by any of the other residents?
First, talk with the nurse staff on the unit, especially the charge nurse or head nurse. Many times changes can be made that will resolve the problem, including a possible room change. If this does not work or the staff is not attentive to your request, speak with the facility's administrator.

35. Is it possible to transfer my relative to a closer or better nursing home?

It is always possible to transfer to another nursing home but many facilities may give preference to people needing first time placement from an acute hospital setting. Many facilities may have a waiting list for transfers. Always speak to the social worker so he or she may advise you on how to make this transition as smooth as possible (see Question #4 also).

36. What do the nursing homes mean when they speak of a "restraint policy?"

Facilities may have varying guidelines regarding when restraints may be placed on a resident (waist, belts or certain types of chairs; see Chapter 4). Some nursing homes now have a "restraint-free" environment in which no restraints of any type are used. The admission coordinator at the nursing home can tell you of the current restraint policy of the facility.

37. Why do nursing homes only allow visiting hours at certain times? Do they ever make exceptions in case my work schedule does not coincide with these times?

All nursing homes have certain visiting hours to allow the staff adequate time and privacy to give required medications, treatments and attend to other personal hygiene needs. Talk with the social worker or the administrator about arranging special times as the standard visitation hours can often be altered for legitimate family schedule conflicts.

38. Can I prevent certain individuals who I feel may disturb my relative, from visiting the nursing home?

Discuss this matter with the nursing staff. Also, do not hesitate to bring your concerns to the attention of the doctor and the administrator. The nursing home is obligated to follow any state regulations regarding the barring of visitors. It is important to note that proper written authorization from the resident or legal next-of-kin is required to bar any individuals from visiting.

39. Is it true that major tranquilizers (antipsychotics and other sedatives) are still used extensively in nursing homes for "noisy" of "annoying" residents?

Only a doctor (or in many states a nurse practitioner or physician assistant) can order such medications and only for specific reasons. Federal regulations now limit the use of such medications in nursing home residents (see Chapter 4). Feel free to discuss your concerns with your relative's doctor.

40. Can I request a special area, room or floor in the nursing home for my relative?

At the time of admission you may certainly request a special area, floor or room but there is often little flexibility in moving individuals around within a nursing home to accommodate everyone's requests. Certain areas within a nursing home may be designated for specific types of residents depending on their overall care needs and this may limit your ability to choose a particular area. Many nursing homes may have a waiting list for families with special requests (e.g., a private room) which the social worker can advise you on.

41. Do residents have an opportunity to request special diets or foods? Can I bring in my relative's favorite foods from time to time? Is a dietitian on staff?

Ask the unit charge nurse about any special requests you have. You may also make an appointment to meet with the dietitian to discuss any concerns you have regarding the food being served at the facility. The doctor will be the one ordering the diet so touch base with him or her if you have concerns in this area. Most nursing homes will allow you to bring in favorite foods for a relative from time to time, especially if their appetite is poor. However, some residents may have specific dietary restrictions and all foods, snacks or desserts must fall within the ordered guidelines, unless a specific exception has been ordered by the doctor. Alcoholic products may only be consumed by residents with a doctor's order so you will need to request this if your relative desires an alcoholic beverage (the amount that can be given at any one time is also written into the order). The nursing staff will be able to advise you what the nursing home's outside food policy currently is. Also, try to work with the nurses to avoid potential problems or conflicts with the facility's established food schedule and rules (e.g., don't try to sneak in prohibited foods, snacks, desserts or alcohol).

42. Do nursing homes allow residents to go outside in nice weather?
Spending time outside is an important change in a resident's routine and should be encouraged. Ask if the home has any special restrictions and find out how the residents are accompanied or supervised while outside. Make sure your relative has the proper clothing to wear outside for the current season. Hats and suntan lotion should be used during periods of hot weather to limit sun exposure and potential dehydration.

43. Can I bring my relative's radio, television and favorite furniture for their room? Are telephones available in the rooms?
Most facilities do not object to audiovisual equipment, assuming this will not deprive a roommate of their space. Some states have strict safety restrictions that may preclude bringing in certain electrical appliances. The facility will be able to assist you with any questions or concerns you may have. However, allowing the resident to keep personal belongings in the room may help reduce the trauma of relocating to a new environment.

All facilities have pay phones on the premises, although they may be in locations not close to your relative's room. Most facilities should allow you to install private phones, although you will be expected to pay all associated costs, rental fees and long distance charges. Telephone installation and service charges are not routinely part of the monthly room and board fee.

44. Do the better nursing homes always cost more money?
Comparison shopping to determine the best value for the dollar is important. Better nursing homes often have a more pleasing physical environment, specialized services, better staffing ratios, equipment in good working order and a reduced employee turnover rate. To maintain such quality, they must often charge a higher daily rate to cover salaries, services and environmental maintenance. Always compare rates between nursing homes, as some excellent homes do have rates that are lower than others. However, the monthly charge should never be the sole factor used in determining the quality of a facility. Remember survey results, which the facility must provide for you at your request, should also be reviewed to obtain a better understanding of the overall care being provided and any areas where future improvement may be required.

45. Is there a list of the best nursing homes?

While some nursing homes have Joint Commission on Accreditation of Healthcare Organizations (JCAHO) approval, there is no national or regional ranking of homes. JCAHO approval usually indicates strict standards have been met, although currently such nursing homes are only inspected every three years (future surveys may be done every eighteen months). However, many excellent nursing homes do not have JCAHO approval. All states now maintain a list of deficiencies that have been found in nursing homes during the most recent inspections and can be obtained at the individual nursing home. Some states may also have this information available on a web page. However, many of these deficiencies are minor in nature (e.g., a mirror in a bathroom was mounted at the wrong angle for a person in a wheelchair to see himself properly) and do not present any real danger to the residents. Other, more serious, deficiencies that jeopardize the health of residents are potentially more dangerous in nature and are specifically listed as such in the posted deficiency list. Remember, a personal tour, interviewing staff and other family members and reviewing facility policies remain the most effective ways of obtaining current information on the care being delivered at any particular facility.

46. What do I do or to whom do I talk to if I feel my relative isn't being cared for properly?

Always speak to the staff nurse first, preferably on the day shift. Then speak with the head nurse or charge nurse. If you are unhappy with their response or solution, call your relative's doctor. He or she may have some control in getting things changed. If both of these attempts to resolve a concern fail, talk with the nursing home administrator. Nursing homes are also obligated to post information on how to reach state officials and the ombudsman assigned to that home (see Chapter 6).

47. Is the total number of beds in a nursing home facility a factor to be considered in selection?

A larger nursing home may be able to provide more activities or other specialized services. Smaller homes, though, may often have a more "home-like" environment. Again, you must be comfortable with the nursing home prior to arranging admission. Consider all aspects of the environment, geographical location, recreational, activities, religious services available and staffing in your decision.

48. Is it important to check out a nursing home with my own doctor?
It is often very helpful to discuss a nursing home with your relative's doctor or your own doctor even if they themselves do not attend at nursing homes. They may have very useful information on the quality of the facility or which doctor on staff at the nursing home they would suggest you select for your relative's doctor. Consider this information when making a decision.

49. How do I find out if the safety procedures of the facility are adequate?
Look for clearly marked safety exits that are unobstructed and not locked. Are hallways wide enough to allow safe passage in an emergency? Are emergency evacuation plans posted on the wall? Ask the social worker how often fire drills and emergency preparedness drills are carried out. Also, ask the admissions coordinator if they have received any deficiencies on state inspections for safety violations in the past two years and, if so, have they been corrected.

50. What do I do if the currently assigned roommate does not interact well with my relative?
Often a family will discover their relative has been assigned to a room with a agitated, "noisy," extremely ill or otherwise incompatible roommate. While few people can afford the luxury of a private room, there are ways of dealing with the problem. The first solution is to talk with the charge nurse and try to obtain a clearer picture of the roommate's prognosis or chances of improvement. If someone has been screaming all night for two years, it is unlikely things will change quickly. If you are unhappy with the choice, speak up! While no family would ideally want this person for a roommate, finding a more appropriate roommate may be possible. Discuss this with the unit charge nurse and social worker.

Appendices

Appendix A

Resident Rights and Responsibilities: A Summary of Federally Mandated Rights for Residents of Nursing Homes

Payment for Services
You have the right to:

- Be fully informed of the services available in the nursing home. If you are paying for the cost of your care we must inform you of the daily rate and charges for any services not covered by that rate. If your care is paid for by Medicare or Medicaid, we must inform you of the services not covered by Medicare or Medicaid and the charges for such services.
- Be informed when there is a change in the charges for items and services.
- Be informed of how to apply for and use Medicare and Medicaid and how to receive refunds for previous payments covered by these programs.
- You cannot be required to waive any rights you may have to receive Medicare or Medicaid, or to give assurance that you are not eligible for or will not apply for Medicare or Medicaid, as a condition of admission to or continued residence in the nursing home.
- You cannot be required to have a third party guarantee payment for your care as a condition of admission to or continued residence in the nursing home.

- If you are eligible for Medicaid assistance, you cannot be required to pay or give the nursing home any gift, money, donation or other consideration as a condition of admission to or continued residence in the nursing home.

Personal Funds
You have the right to:

- Manage your personal financial affairs and cannot be required to deposit your personal funds with the nursing home.
- Have the nursing home manage your personal funds if you authorize this in writing. You have the right to a quarterly accounting of your funds. A separate statement about how the nursing home manages resident's funds may be provided to you.

Note! Each state may also establish certain other rights.

Care
You have the right to:

- Choose your personal attending physician (doctor). The nursing home may require you to use another doctor if your doctor does not comply with all applicable statutes or regulations.
- Be fully informed, in a language you understand, about your total health status, including your medical condition.
- Be fully informed in advance about care and treatment and any changes in your care and treatment that may affect your well-being.
- Refuse treatment including life support systems, in accordance with state law. If the nursing home is unwilling to honor your wishes regarding the use of life support systems, it must attempt to transfer you to a nursing home that will honor your wishes.
- Participate in planning care and treatment or changes in care and treatment unless you are unable to as defined by state law.
- Administer your own drugs, if your care planning team determines that it would be safe for you to do so.
- Refuse to participate in experimental research.

Treatment
You have the right to:

- Be free from verbal, sexual, physical or mental abuse, corporal punishment and involuntary seclusion.
- Be free from restraints administered for discipline or convenience and that are not required to treat your medical symptoms. Physical and chemical restraints may be used only to ensure your physical safety or enable you to function better, and then only on the written order of a doctor, except in an emergency. The doctor's order must state when and for how long the restraints are to be used.
- Have psychoactive drugs, antipsychotics, antidepressants, anti-anxieties or hypnotic-sedative medications administered only on the order of a doctor. The drug will be administered as part of a written care plan designed to eliminate or modify the symptoms the drug was prescribed to treat, and only if an independent external consultant reviews whether your drug plan is appropriate at least once a year.
- Not perform work at the nursing home. If you choose to perform work for the nursing home, your care plan must state your need or desire to work, the type of work you are performing, that you are performing work as a volunteer or for payment at prevailing rates and that you agree with the plan.

Personal and Clinical Records
You have the right to:

- Privacy and confidentiality regarding all records kept by the nursing home pertaining to you.
- Approve or refuse the release of these records to anyone outside the nursing home, except when you are transferred to another health care institution or the release of records is required by law.
- Access all records pertaining to you within twenty-four hours of your request or the request of your legal representative.
- Purchase photocopies of your records after you have inspected them. The nursing home must provide them to you within two working days of your request.

Transfer and Discharge
You have the right to:

- Be allowed to stay in the nursing home and may not be discharged from the nursing home, except as provided for by state and federal law.
- Appeal an involuntary transfer or discharge from the nursing home.

Federal and state law permit an involuntary transfer or discharge when:

- It is necessary for your welfare and your welfare cannot be met in the nursing home.
- It is appropriate because your health has improved so that you no longer need the services provided by the nursing home.
- The health or safety of individuals in the nursing home is endangered.
- Your account remains in arrears after a reasonable effort has been made to collect the amount due.
- The nursing home ceases to operate.
- You must be given thirty days notice of a transfer or discharge from the nursing home unless:
  - The transfer or discharge is made because the health or safety of individuals in the nursing home is endangered.
  - Your health has improved significantly to allow for a more immediate transfer or discharge.
  - You have resided in the nursing home for less than 30 days.

In such cases, you must be given as much notice as practicable. You may be involuntarily transferred from one room to another within the nursing home only for medical reasons or for your welfare or that of other patients as documented in your medical record, or, if you receiving Medicaid assistance, from a private to a semi-private room (two or more beds). You must be given written notice as stated above.

If only part of the nursing home is certified for participation in the Medicare program (a "Medicare distinct part"), you may refuse transfer into or out of the Medicare distinct part. Refusing a transfer will not affect your entitlement or eligibility for Medicare or Medicaid.

Visits
You have the right to:

- Be visited by your family.
- Be visited by your doctor, by the long-term-care ombudsman and representatives of federal and state agencies concerned with patient care.
- Be visited by other persons of your choice, including persons who provide health, social or legal services to patients residing in a skilled nursing home subject to reasonable restrictions.
- Refuse to receive any visitor you do not want to see.

Group Activities
You have the right to:

- Participate in social, religious and community activities that do not interfere with the rights of other patients.
- Organize and participate in patient groups in the nursing home.
- Meet with families of other patients in the nursing home.

Grievances
You have the right to:

- Voice grievances without discrimination or reprisal.
- Have prompt efforts made by the nursing home to resolve any grievances you may have, including those about the behavior of other patients.
- File a complaint with any state agency regarding abuse, neglect, misappropriation of patients' property or noncompliance with advance directive requirements. A list of the names, addresses and telephone numbers of these and other agencies you may to contact can be obtained from the nursing home.

Privacy
You have the right to:

- Privacy in accommodations and in receiving personal and medical care and treatment.
- Privacy in visits and in meetings with family and patient groups.
- Associate and communicate privately with persons of your choice, including other residents.
- Privacy for visits with your spouse.
- Share a room with your spouse if he or she is a patient of the same nursing home subject to his or her consent and if such a room is available.
- The nursing home is not required to provide you with a private room.

Communicating with Others
You have the right to:

- Privacy in written and spoken communications.
- Send and promptly receive unopened mail.
- Have stationery, stamps and writing implements made available by the nursing home for you to purchase.
- Reasonable access to a telephone that you can use without being overheard.
- Receive information from agencies that act as patient advocates and to have the opportunity to contact such agencies.
- Know where to find, and to see, the results of current federal, state and local inspection reports and plans of correction.

Exercising Your Rights
You have the right to:

- Exercise your rights as a patient and as a citizen or resident of the United States.
- Be treated equally with other patients in receiving care and services and regarding transfer and discharge, regardless of the source of payment for your care.

- Exercise your rights without fear of discrimination, interference, coercion or reprisal.
- If you are incapable of exercising your rights, a representative designated in accordance with state law exercise your rights on your behalf.

Notice of Rights and Services
You have the right to:

- Be fully informed, orally and in writing, in a language you understand, of your rights and the nursing home's rules governing your conduct and responsibilities.
- Be notified of changes in your rights and in the nursing home's rules.

Dignity and Self-Determination
You have the right to:

- Be treated with consideration, respect and full recognition of your dignity and individuality.
- Reasonable accommodation of your individual needs and preferences, except when your health or safety or the health or safety of others would be endangered.
- Choose activities, schedules and health care consistent with your interests and your plan of care.
- Make choices about aspects of your life that are significant to you.
- Keep and use your personal possessions, as space permits, unless doing so would infringe on the rights, health or safety of other patients.
- Receive notice before your roommate is changed.

Appendix B

Contact Information for State Ombudsman Offices

Telephone Numbers

Alabama	334-242-5743
Alaska	907-334-4480
Arizona	602-542-6440
Arkansas	501-682-2441
California	916-324-3968
Colorado	800-288-1376
Connecticut	860-424-5200
Delaware	302-577-4791
District of Columbia (Washington, DC)	202-434-2140
Florida	888-831-0404
Georgia	888-454-5826
Hawaii	808-586-0100

Idaho	877-471-2777
Illinois	217-785-3143
Indiana	800-545-7763
Iowa	515-242-3327
Kansas	785-296-3017
Kentucky	800-373-2991
Louisiana	225-342-1700
Maine	800-499-0229
Maryland	410-767-1100
Massachusetts	617-727-7750
Michigan	866-485-9393
Minnesota	800-657-3591
Missouri	573-526-0727
Mississippi	601-359-4929
Montana	800-551-3191
Nebraska	402-471-2307
Nevada	775-688-2964
New Hampshire	603-271-4375
New Jersey	609-943-4026

New Mexico	505-255-0971
New York	518-474-0108
North Carolina	919-733-8395
North Dakota	800-451-8693
Ohio	614-644-7922
Oklahoma	405-521-6734
Oregon	503-378-6533
Pennsylvania	717-783-7247
Puerto Rico	787-725-1515
Rhode Island	401-785-3340
South Carolina	800-868-9095
South Dakota	866-854-5465
Tennessee	615-741-2056
Texas	800-252-2412
Utah	801-538-3924
Vermont	802-863-5620
Virginia	804-644-2804
Washington	253-838-6810
West Virginia	304-558-3317

Wisconsin   800-815-0015

Wyoming   307-322-5553

Appendix C

Glossary

Accredited facility
A nursing home or other healthcare organization accredited by the Joint Commission on the Accreditation of Healthcare Organizations (JCAHO). Accreditation is achieved only after the facility passes a thorough inspection and it is time-limited (usually between eighteen months and three years). It is not the same as the state licensing procedure for nursing homes.

Activities of daily living (ADLs)
This term refers to those activities related to self-care issues such as feeding, grooming, bathing, toileting, ambulation and dressing. These services must be provided by nursing home staff to any resident requiring help.

Acute care
A setting where advanced lifesaving , surgical or other medical interventions can be delivered; usually implies a general hospital setting. Acute care settings may also include intensive care units and emergency department locations.

Adult daycare
Social, psychological and medical services provided to physically or mentally challenged individuals in a nonresidential setting during daytime hours. Usually only open Monday through Friday.

Allowable cost
The maximum daily reimbursable fee paid by the state for recipients of Medicaid. Medicaid in many states restricts certain medications (e.g.,

over-the-counter products) or services (e.g., limited podiatry and dental coverage). Medicare also has allowable costs for all covered services.

Alzheimer's disease

The common form of dementia which leads to progressive loss of brain function and the ability to care for one's self. It is progressive and not curable, although medications exist that allow for successful treatment for many of the common symptoms that can develop (e.g., depression, insomnia and cognitive worsening).

Annual survey

The process of inspecting the nursing home by the state to see ensure it meets all applicable state and federal regulations and rules regarding the care being delivered to the residents.

Assistive device

A tool, prosthesis or adaptive aid that helps an individual compensate for certain physical disabilities (e.g., hearing aids, eyeglasses, canes and wheelchairs).

Attending physician

The doctor of record for your loved one who is responsible for the overall plan of care and the prescribing of all medications. A nurse practitioner or physician assistant may work under the direction of a physician.

Bed-bound or bed-fast

Refers to a medical condition in which one is confined to bed and cannot ambulate or get out of the bed without assistance. Any transfers out of the bed will require the help of one or two certified nursing assistants or other staff or the use of a device called a mechanical lift.

Behavioral interventions

Non-pharmaceutical (medication) actions to defuse an acute emotional or physical outburst. For example, a staff nurse separates two arguing residents and moves them to different locations on the ward. Also, a resident who is becoming agitated because of a particular program on the television will be moved to a more quite place on the unit.

Case-mix payments

A reimbursement system based on the theory that payment for long-term care services should be based on the illness or special needs of each resident. Due to the requirement that all residents are assessed on a regular basis, it is possible to determine the average resident profile for each facility. This average profile is then used to determine the average daily payment to the facility by the state under Medicaid.

Catheter

A flexible plastic tube inserted through the urethra and into the bladder to assist with urine drainage.

Certificate of need

Many states require that new nursing home construction be justified by filing what is known as a "certificate of need" based on the estimated demand for long-term care (nursing home) beds within a certain geographic area. A state often controls the number of nursing homes in the state by limiting the number of new certificates approved. No nursing homes in the United States can be built without first having obtained an approved certificate of need.

Charge nurse

An LPN or RN who is assigned the responsibility over the staff and residents of a unit of a nursing home for the shift (usually eight hours in length). A charge nurse is on-site during the time they are carrying out this function and such a designated person is available each shift, seven days a week.

CNA (certified nursing assistant) or nurse's aide

An individual who has received a minimum of seventy-five hours of classroom and on-site training to learn how to feed, transfer, groom and attend to other needs of nursing home residents. This individual does much of the "hands on" care being delivered and works under the supervision of a nurse. This certification must be maintained by the CNA obtaining a certain number of hours of inservice education and is renewed on a regular basis.

Centers for Medicare and Medicaid (CMS)

The federal program that administers the Medicare and Medicaid programs that cover much of nursing home care, including the inspection and enforcement of rules and regulations.

Complaint visit

A term that refers to a visit to a nursing home made by a state surveyor in response to a complaint made about the facility to the appropriate state agency by a resident, family member or visitor. An investigation is conducted to either validate or refute the complaint.

Contractures

Shortening of the tendons and muscles of a limb causing either the knees, arms, hands or feet to curl up. This condition can often be prevented or treated by physical therapy but if often permanent in nature and due to the late effects from a stroke or dementia.

Custodial care

A term that refers to the chronic care given to a long-term resident of a nursing facility. This term encompasses all of the feeding, ambulation, dressing, medication administration, grooming, toileting and monitoring that an individual requires each day and is carried out by the staff members of the nursing home.

Decertification of participation (termination)

This is the most severe of the available penalties that a state agency can impose on a nursing home and involves the formal revocation of a facility's ability to participate in the Medicare and Medicaid programs. This decertification also prevents the admission of new residents to the facility if they are entitled to receive Medicare or Medicaid benefits.

Decubitus ulcers (pressure ulcers or pressure sores)

This is the old term for any breakdown in the surface of the skin due to unrelieved pressure (also once known as "bed sores"). They may be aggravated by malnutrition, dehydration, anemia, failing to turn a bedbound individual on a regular basis or other medical factors. The current term that is used is "pressure ulcers."

Deficiencies

The term that refers to deviations from the applicable standard of care that are detected during a survey visit. The facility is obligated to address and correct all deficiencies if they wish to avoid monetary fines or termination from Medicare and Medicaid participation. Although not all deficiencies are life-threatening to residents, all must be corrected within a time-specified period.

Dementia

Refers to the loss of intellectual function and may be due to Alzheimer's disease, vascular processes, strokes or other etiologies.

Diagnosis-related groups (DRGs)

A classification system that groups illnesses to a four or five digit numerical code. It is often the basis for reimbursement by a variety of insurance payors in the acute hospital setting.

Dietitian

A state-registered individual with special training in nutrition who is responsible for the overall nutritional needs of every resident in a nursing home.

Discharge

The formal releasing of a resident from a nursing facility to another site. All discharges must be approved by the attending physician and an order given.

Distinct part

A term referring to a specified portion or wing of a nursing home that can provide special services to a resident (e.g., a subacute unit providing Medicare-reimbursed daily physical therapy).

Director of nursing (DON)

Refers to the person who is the director of nursing, the individual directly in charge of all licensed and allied nursing personnel in the nursing home. Often controls hiring and firing of nursing employees and is often involved in dealing with family concerns.

Dually certified facility

A nursing home that is legally able to offer both Medicare and Medicaid services to residents residing in any such designated beds.

Feeding tube

A plastic or rubber tube inserted through the nose (naso-gastric) or the stomach wall (percutaneous endoscopic gastrostomy—PEG—tube) that allows nutrition and water to be administered to someone who is not able to orally take adequate food and water.

Follow-up visit

A term that either refers to the monthly or bimonthly visits made by the attending physician or a brief return visit by a state survey agency in order to determine a facility's progress on correcting any deficiencies noted on a previous survey inspection.

Functional impairment

The inability on the part of a resident to perform functions such as dressing, using the toilet, eating, bathing or ambulation.

Geri Chair

A high-backed cushioned recliner-like chair with an associated leg and foot rest. It can be moved around on wheels by staff but can not be self-propelled like a wheelchair. As the individual placed in such a device can often not get out of it without assistance, it is classified as a restraint and can only be used on the order of a physician.

Healthcare provider

Any physician ("M.D."), dentist, nurse practitioner, physician assistant, podiatrist, psychologist, psychiatrist (also an M.D.) licensed to provide care in a nursing-home setting.

Heavy-care resident

A term that refers to nursing home residents who require a great deal of "hands-on" care during the day. These individuals usually have a significant degree of functional impairment and often have advanced stages of dementia and are bed-bound. A facility would prefer not to have a high number of heavy-care residents as the staffing pattern is usually designed to handle a more balanced "case mix" of residents.

HIPAA (Health Insurance Portability and Accountability Act)

This is the new comprehensive series of federal regulations protecting healthcare privacy. HIPAA provides individuals with broad protections regarding the confidentiality of their health information. Compliance with all aspects of the HIPAA is required of all organizations that maintain or transmit electronic health information and failure to comply with the rules can result in severe civil and criminal penalties. These rules took effect in April of 2003.

Incontinence

The inability to control bowel or bladder function (or both) and is often seen as a complication of strokes and dementia. Treatment protocols exist for this clinical problem.

JCAHO

See **Accredited facility**.

Key indicators

These refer to measures of quality of care and quality of life which focus on care given to nursing home residents. The federal government has established a number of key indicators (currently about forty-five for long-term care and post-acute care services) for each nursing home that can be tracked on the Internet by going to their web page (www.cms.gov).

Level of care

The amount of medical and nursing care that any individual nursing home resident requires. This level can alter over time as an individual's medical condition changes. A "skilled level of care" refers to a higher requirement than "custodial care."

Licensed practical nurse (LPN) or licensed vocational nurse (LVN)

An individual who has received a minimum of eighteen months of training in the field of nursing. Supervises the CNAs in their daily activities.

Such a nurse is present on every shift (usually eight hours long) at the nursing home, every day of the week.

Medicaid

A state program (with certain federal subsidies) authorized by Title XIX of the Social Security Act and which provides reimbursement for all bed costs, medications and physician fees for those nursing home residents who otherwise do not have the means to pay for such care. Each state (with the exception of Arizona) has their own specific income guidelines for eligibility for acceptance of an individual into the Medicaid program.

Medical director

The physician required under federal regulations to oversee all medical and nursing care being delivered at a nursing home. Although the federal Omnibus Budget Reconciliation Act (OBRA) regulations (see **OBRA**) place great responsibility on this position, no specific enforcement powers are given. The medical director is required to be available twenty-four hours a day, seven days a week, to arrange for emergency medical intervention if the attending physician of record cannot be located. Facility staff should always be able to reach their medical director or the assigned covering medical director if they have an issue that cannot be resolved through other means.

Medicare

A federally funded health insurance program authorized by Title XVIII of the Social Security Act to pay for medical care for older and disabled beneficiaries. Medicare will pay for up to 100 days of post-acute (post-hospitalization) stay in a subacute (post-acute care) unit in a nursing home if the facility participates in the program. There are specific requirements for post-acute care coverage (e.g., minimum of a three-day acute hospital stay and the ongoing need for daily medical, physical, speech or occupational therapy) and specific rules of continuation in the program (e.g., must continue to progress towards goals and attend daily sessions) and has time constraints (e.g., no more than 100 days of coverage per calender year within a sixty-day coverage-free interval).

Nurse's aide
See **CNA**.

Nurse practitioner
A licensed registered nurse with advanced training who practices in the nursing home under the supervision (which may be via telephone at times) of the attending physician. He or she is able to directly prescribe certain treatments and medications (the actual scope of their practice authority varies by state).

OBRA
A federal bill from 1987 that established minimum care requirements for all nursing homes in the United States. Certain resident rights were spelled out, including the right to adequate and appropriate medical care, the right to be free from unnecessary physical and chemical restraints and the right to participate in the creation and revision of the care plan (see Appendix A).

Ombusman
A representative of the state agency charged with investigating and resolving complaints made by or on behalf of older individuals who are residents of nursing homes. These individuals advocate for any resident of a nursing home when care concerns arise. These complaints may relate to any activity that can adversely affect the health, safety, welfare and rights of the individual resident. Each state is mandated to have an ombudsman program, although much of the actual work is contracted out to local agencies.

Out-of-pocket expenditures
This refers to any amount of money that must be paid by the resident or their family for any non-covered services.

Resident Care Plan or Care Plan
A care plan developed by members of an interdisciplinary team in conjunction with the resident or the family member, to review the medical, nursing and psychosocial issues that a resident faces during their stay in a

nursing facility. The care plan is reviewed on a quarterly basis or sooner if an individual's medical condition changes.

Physician's assistant
A licensed individual who has attended a prescribed college curriculum, generally at the masters degree level, and who practices in the nursing home under the supervision (which may be via telephone at times) of the attending physician. He or she is able to directly prescribe certain treatments and medications (the actual scope of their practice authority varies by state).

Range-of-motion exercises
Movement of the limbs and muscles by a staff member or physical therapist to maintain or restore strength or flexibility and to prevent or treat contractures.

Rehabilitation
Those special services (e.g., speech, occupational and physical therapy) that are used to restore, if possible, an individual's overall functional level to their baseline.

Resource utilization groups
A standardized method of grouping nursing home residents with the specific services they require during their stay.

Skilled nursing facility
A nursing home licensed by the state to provide specialized skilled nursing services such as intravenous therapy, pressure ulcer care, or monitoring certain medication effects.

Spend-down
Under Medicaid regulations, the method by which a resident (or their legal representative) arranges to utilize ("spend") any existing cash assets, stocks, bonds and other insurance coverage (e.g., Medicare) until such time as they qualify for Medicaid eligibility.

Staff-resident ratio

The number of staff members present on any given shift and their assigned number of residents.

"Stat"

Refers to any test or procedure ordered on an emergency basis by the healthcare provider.

Twenty-four-hour nursing care

A resident who, because of their medical conditions and nursing requirements, must have the presence of a licensed nurse (LPN or RN) twenty-four hours per day in the nursing home setting.

Appendix D

A Checklist of Twenty-Five Items to Observe When You Visit a Nursing Home

1. Does the facility appear clean?

2. Is respect and compassion shown to all of the residents, regardless of their mental abilities?

3. Is privacy provided during all personal care treatments?

4. Is confidentiality of medical information evident in the facility?

5. Is your loved one's outer clothing clean and neat appearing?

6. Is proper grooming and oral hygiene for your loved one evident?

7. Do you get your questions answered in a timely manner?

8. Does the food appear appetizing and is it served at a proper temperature? Are meals served on time?

9. Is sufficient time given for meals to be eaten?

10. Is adequate staff available every day of the week to help feed those residents requiring assistance?

11. Is adequate staffing present when you visit to perform routine care and administer medications?

12. Does turnover among staff members appear to be relatively low?

13. Is the staff member assigned to your loved one relatively constant and familiar with the ordered care plan?

14. Is toileting done in a timely and respectful manner?

15. Is the call bell answered promptly (less than five minutes)?

16. Are linen changes for the bed done as required?

17. Is adequate fluid present in the room and within reach?

18. Do you know who the doctor or nurse practitioner for your loved one is and how to contact him yourself if necessary?

19. Is the facility free of unpleasant odors?

20. Are there adequate and stimulating activities scheduled on a daily basis in the nursing home, including weekends?

21. Do staff members demonstrate an appropriate level of friendliness and respect for all of the visitors?

22. Are the rooms kept clean and functioning properly by personnel in the housekeeping and maintenance departments?

23. Do both the administrator and director of nursing appear to be approachable and concerned with any issues you may have regarding care practices in the facility?

24. Is bathing or showering performed on a proper schedule so it does not disturb the sleep cycle of your relative?

25. Is the facility free of environmental hazards such as wet floors or articles on the floor that may cause trips or falls?

Appendix E

Agencies and Sources for Information and Referrals

Alzheimer's Association
919 North Michigan Ave., Suite 1100
Chicago, IL 60611
800-272-3900
www.alz.org

American Association for Geriatric Psychiatry
7910 Woodmont Ave., Suite 1050
Bethesda, MD 20814
301-654-7850
www.aagpga.org

American Geriatrics Society
350 5th Ave., Suite 801
New York, NY 10118
212-308-1414
www.americangeriatrics.org
Note: National organization of physicians active in geriatric care and teaching

The American Medical Directors Association
10480 Little Patuxent Parkway, Suite 760
Columbia, MD 21044
410-740-9743
www.amda.com
Note: National organization of nursing home medical directors

American Society of Consultant Pharmacists
1321 Duke St.
Alexandria, VA 22314
703-739-1316
www.ascp.com

Coalition to Protect America's Elders
8094 Buck Lake Rd.
Tallahassee, FL 32311
850-216-2727

Centers for Medicare and Medicaid Services (CMS)
7500 Security Blvd.
Baltimore, MD 21244
877-267-2323
410-786-3000
www.cms.gov

National Association for Continence
P.O.Box 8310
Spartanburg, SC 29305
800-252-3337
www.nafc.org
Note: Info on incontinence issues and their treatment

National Citizens' Coalition for Nursing Home Reform (NCCNHR)
1424 16th St., NW #202
Washington, DC 20036
202-332-2275
www.nursinghomeaction.org

National Committee for the Prevention of Elder Abuse
c/o Institute on Aging, Medical Center of Central Massachusetts
111 Belmont St.
Worcester, MA 01605
508-793-6166

National Institute on Aging
U.S. Department of Health and Human Services
Public Health Service
800-222-2225
www.nia.nih.gov
Note: various publications related to aging

National Hospice and Palliative Care Organization
1700 Diagonal Rd., Suite 330
Alexandria, CA 22314
800-658-8898
www.nhpco.org
Note: Information on end-of-life issues

National Stroke Association
9707 East Easter Lane
Englewood, CO 80112
800-787-6537
www.stroke.org

Additional Resources

*Caregiver's Reprive: A Guide to Emotional Survival When You're
Caring for Someone You Love*
Aurene L. Brandt, PhD
Impact Publishers
P.O. Box 6016
Atascadero, CA 93423

Nursing Homes: Getting Good Care There
Sarah Greene Burget et al.
National Citizens' Coalition for Nursing Home Reform (NCCNHR)
1424 16th St. NW, #202
Washington, DC 20036
202-332-2275
www.nursinghomeaction.org

About the Author

Dr. Andrew Weinberg is currently Professor of Clinical Medicine at the University of South Carolina School of Medicine and Director of Geriatrics and Extended Care at the Dorn VA Medical Center in Columbia, SC. He has previously held faculty appointments at the Yale School of Medicine, Harvard Medical School, Mayo Medical School and the Emory University School of Medicine.

Dr. Weinberg is also the current chairman of the Special Interest Group on Long-Term Care of the American Geriatrics Society in New York and a member of the Public Policy Committee of the American Medical Directors Association. He is also the current president of the South Carolina Geriatrics Society. In his free time, Dr. Weinberg serves as a Reserve Naval Flight Surgeon assigned to a Marine Corps helicopter squadron out of Norfolk, Virginia.

Index